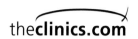

ORTHOPEDIC CLINICS

OF NORTH AMERICA

The Treatment of
Unicompartmental Arthritis
of the Knee

GUEST EDITOR
Jack M. Bert, MD

October 2005 • Volume 36 • Number 4

SAUNDERS

An Imprint of Elsevier, Inc.
PHILADELPHIA   LONDON   TORONTO   MONTREAL   SYDNEY   TOKYO

W.B. SAUNDERS COMPANY
A Division of Elsevier Inc.

Elsevier Inc., 1600 John F. Kennedy Blvd., Suite 1800, Philadelphia, PA 19103-2899.

http://www.orthopedic.theclinics.com

ORTHOPEDIC CLINICS OF NORTH AMERICA   Volume 36, Number 4
October 2005   ISSN 0030-5898
Editor: Debora Dellapena   ISBN 1-4160-2747-5

The ideas and opinions expressed in *Orthopedic Clinics of North America* do not necessarily reflect those of the Publisher. The Publisher does not assume any responsibility for any injury and/or damage to persons or property arising out of or related to any use of the material contained in this periodical. The reader is advised to check the appropriate medical literature and the product information currently provided by the manufacturer of each drug to be administered to verify the dosage, the method and duration of administration, or contraindications. It is the responsibility of the treating physician or other health care professional, relying on independent experience and knowledge of the patient, to determine drug dosages and the best treatment for the patient. Mention of any product in this issue should not be construed as endorsement by the contributors, editors, or the Publisher of the product or manufacturers' claims.

Orthopedic Clinics of North America (ISSN 0030-5898) is published quarterly (For Post Office use only: Volume 36 issue 4 of 4) by Elsevier Inc. Corporate and editorial offices: Elsevier Inc., 1600 John F. Kennedy Blvd., Suite 1800, Philadelphia, PA 19103-2899. Accounting and circulation offices: 6277 Sea Harbor Drive, Orlando, FL 33887-4800. Periodicals postage paid at Orlando, FL 32862, and additional mailing offices. Subscription prices are $190.00 per year for (US individuals), $315.00 per year for (US institutions), $225.00 per year (Canadian individuals), $370.00 per year (Canadian institutions), $260.00 per year (international individuals), $370.00 per year (international institutions), $95.00 per year (US students), $130.00 per year (Canadian and international students). Foreign air speed delivery is included in all *Clinics* subscription prices. All prices are subject to change without notice. POSTMASTER: Send address changes to *Orthopedic Clinics of North America*, W.B. Saunders Company, Periodicals Fulfillment, Orlando, FL 32887-4800. **Customer Service: 1-800-654-2452 (US). From outside of the US, call 1-407-345-4000. E-mail: hhspcs@harcourt.com.**

Reprints. For copies of 100 or more, of articles in this publication, please contact the Commercial Reprints Department, Elsevier Inc., 360 Park Avenue South, New York, New York 10010-1710. Tel. (212) 633-3813 Fax: (212) 462-1935 e-mail: reprints@elsevier.com

Orthopedic Clinics of North America is covered in *Index Medicus, Cinahl, Excerpta Medica,* and *Cumulative Index to Nursing and Allied Health Literature.*

Printed in the United States of America.

GUEST EDITOR

JACK M. BERT, MD, FACS, Summit Orthopedics, Ltd., St. Paul; Adjunct Clinical Professor, University of Minnesota School of Medicine, Minneapolis, Minnesota

CONTRIBUTORS

WINSLOW ALFORD, MD, West Bay Orthopedics, Warwick, Rhode Island

ANNUNZIATO AMENDOLA, MD, Professor of Orthopaedic Surgery, Department of Orthopaedics, University of Iowa; Director, Sports Medicine Center, University of Iowa Hospitals and Clinics, Iowa City, Iowa

F. ALAN BARBER, MD, FACS, Plano Orthopedic and Sports Medicine Center, Plano, Texas

JACK M. BERT, MD, FACS, Summit Orthopedics, Ltd., St. Paul; Adjunct Clinical Professor, University of Minnesota School of Medicine, Minneapolis, Minnesota

PAUL E. CALDWELL III, MD, Fellow, Mississippi Sports Medicine and Orthopaedic Center, University of Mississippi School of Medicine, Jackson, Mississippi

BRIAN J. COLE, MD, MBA, Associate Professor, Departments of Orthopedics and Anatomy and Cell Biology, and Director, Rush Cartilage Restoration Center, Rush University Medical Center, Chicago, Illinois

DAVID A. COONS, DO, Plano Orthopedic and Sports Medicine Center, Plano, Texas

BRIAN DAY, MD, Associate Professor, Department of Orthopaedics, University of British Columbia, Vancouver, British Columbia; Medical Director, Cambie Surgery Centre, Vancouver, British Columbia

SCOTT D. GILLOGLY, MD, Atlanta Sports Medicine and Orthopaedic Center, Atlanta, Georgia

RICHARD H. HALLOCK, MD, Orthopedic Institute of Pennsylvania, Camp Hill, Pennsylvania

BRYAN T. HANYPSIAK, MD, Orthopaedic Associates of Long Island, East Setauket, New York

BERT R. MANDELBAUM, MD, Santa Monica Orthopaedic and Sports Medicine Group, Santa Monica, California

THOMAS H. MYERS, MD, Atlanta Sports Medicine and Orthopaedic Center, Atlanta, Georgia

LUDOVICO PANARELLA, MD, Fellow, Sports Medicine, Department of Orthopaedics, University of Iowa Hospital and Clinics, Iowa City, Iowa

JASON M. SCOPP, MD, Peninsula Orthopaedic Associates, Salisbury, Maryland

NICHOLAS A. SGAGLIONE, MD, Chief, Division of Sports Medicine, Associate Chairman, Department of Orthopaedics, North Shore University Hospital, Manhasset; Associate Clinical Professor of Surgery, Albert Einstein College of Medicine, Great Neck, New York

BENJAMIN S. SHAFFER, MD, DC Sportsmedicine Institute, Washington, DC

WALTER R. SHELTON, MD, Clinical Instructor, Department of Orthopaedic Surgery, Mississippi Sports Medicine and Orthopaedic Center, University of Mississippi School of Medicine, Jackson, Mississippi

C. THOMAS VANGSNESS, Jr, MD, Professor of Orthopaedic Surgery, Department of Orthopaedic Surgery, Keck School of Medicine, University of Southern California, Los Angeles, California

CONTENTS

> Treatment of the knee with unicompartmental osteoarthritis remains a challenging clinical problem. Despite pharmacologic advances and surgical innovations, the ideal strategy for the patient who has single-compartment degenerative disease can be complicated. The understanding and management of this problem are further confounded by the fact that so much of the data are unreliable. Given these constraints, this article outlines the current alternatives available in nonoperatively managing the symptomatic unicompartmental arthritic knee.

> The evidence supporting the therapeutic value of arthroscopic debridement of the knee is overwhelming. However, there is a need for better-designed clinical trials comparing arthroscopic debridement to established alternative treatments. The most important factor in determining success is proper patient selection, and many who have osteoarthritis of the knee will not benefit from arthroscopic debridement. Patients who have end-stage osteoarthritis or severe malalignment and those who do not have mechanical symptoms are unlikely to improve. The important considerations are how effective the treatment is and whether the expected benefits justify the risks, potential complications, and cost. An objective analysis of outcome studies in patients who have osteoarthritis of the knee joint clearly shows that properly selected patients will benefit greatly from arthroscopic debridement and many will be saved from the increased morbidity and potential complications of alternative treatments.

> The clinical consequences of articular cartilage defects of the knee are pain, swelling, mechanical symptoms, athletic and functional disability, and osteoarthritis. Full thickness articular cartilage defects have a poor capacity to heal. The challenge to restore the articular cartilage surface is multidimensional, faced by basic scientists in the laboratory

and orthopedic surgeons in the operating room. This article provides an overview of the contemporary treatment options available for the restoration of articular cartilage defects of the knee.

Radiofrequency Use on Articular Cartilage Lesions

C. Thomas Vangsness, Jr

The incidence of knee arthritis is increasing in our society and presents many dilemmas to the patient and doctor. Recent advances in arthroscopic treatment of arthritis have lead to the development of radiofrequency energy as an adjunctive tool for many arthroscopic procedures. Of great concern is the recent use of radiofrequency energy to treat articular cartilage lesions in the knee.

Treatment of Full-Thickness Chondral Defects with Autologous Chondrocyte Implantation

Scott D. Gillogly and Thomas H. Myers

Autologous chondrocyte implantation (ACI) is a reproducible treatment option for large full-thickness symptomatic chondral injuries with appropriate knowledge of technique and patient selection. It provides a cellular repair that offers a high percentage of good to excellent clinical results over a long follow-up period. It is applicable over a wide range of chondral injuries from simple to more complex lesions. It is essential that the intra-articular environment be as close to normal as possible for successful cartilage repair. Coexisting knee pathology must be aggressively treated. ACI does have a prolonged postoperative rehabilitation course necessitated by the biologic nature of the repair, and patients must be able to comply with the rehabilitation and temporary restrictions required for a successful outcome.

Arthroscopic Osteochondral Autografting

David A. Coons and F. Alan Barber

Arthroscopic osteochondral autografting is indicated for unipolar, full thickness articular cartilage lesions between 1 and 2.5 cm in diameter. A stable, properly-aligned knee is important to a good outcome. This procedure should not be performed in the presence of generalized osteoarthritis. Arthroscopic osteochondral autografting allows the restoration of hyaline articular cartilage with zonal matching of the graft. It is cost-effective, can be performed on an outpatient basis, and results in durable resurfacing with excellent long-term results.

Indications for Allografts

Paul E. Caldwell III and Walter R. Shelton

Allografts continue to be popular in orthopaedic reconstruction procedures of the knee. Approximately 1 million musculoskeletal allografts were distributed in the United Sates in 2004 alone. Ligament allografts, osteochondral allografts, and meniscal transplants have all demonstrated success in knee reconstructions. The advantages of allograft tissue include the lack of donor site morbidity, shorter operative times, ease of sizing, and a lack of clinically significant immunologic reactions. These advantages should be weighed against the risk for disease transmission, increased cost, and increased time of graft incorporation. Throughout the consent process, comprehensive patient education is imperative to assist in this important decision.

Unicompartmental Knee Replacement 513
Jack M. Bert

Because of the resurgence in popularity of unicompartmental knee arthroplasty, primarily as a result of the mini-incision technique, it is important to understand the advantages and disadvantages of this procedure compared with total knee arthroplasty and upper tibial osteotomy, as well as the indications and contraindications for this procedure.

FORTHCOMING ISSUES

RECENT ISSUES

ORTHOPEDIC
CLINICS
OF NORTH AMERICA

Orthop Clin N Am 36 (2005) xi

Preface

The Treatment of Unicompartmental Arthritis of the Knee

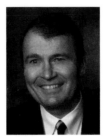

Jack M. Bert, MD
Guest Editor

Unicompartmental arthritis of the knee is extremely common in the middle-aged and older patient. There are multiple treatment modalities available, including nonsurgical conservative care, arthroscopic debridement, varying types of cartilage transplants, osteotomy, and finally, unicompartmental replacement.

An algorithm for the treatment of cartilage defects is presented and multiple articles dealing with these treatment modalities are discussed in detail along with future trends using biologic materials.

It is important to match the appropriate treatment to the patient's age and expectations of each of these procedures. Hopefully, this issue of the *Orthopedic Clinics of North America*, containing multiple articles written by national knee experts, will help enlighten the orthopedic surgeon as to the myriad of options available and the appropriate indications for the treatment of unicompartmental disease of the knee.

Jack M. Bert, MD
Summit Orthopedics, Ltd.
17 West Exchange Street, Suite 307
St. Paul, MN 55102, USA

University of Minnesota School of Medicine
Minneapolis, MN, USA
E-mail address: bertx001@tc.umn.edu

0030-5898/05/$ – see front matter © 2005 Elsevier Inc. All rights reserved.
doi:10.1016/j.ocl.2005.06.002

ELSEVIER
SAUNDERS

Orthop Clin N Am 36 (2005) 401–411

ORTHOPEDIC
CLINICS
OF NORTH AMERICA

Nonoperative Treatment of Unicompartmental Arthritis of the Knee

Bryan T. Hanypsiak, MD[a],*, Benjamin S. Shaffer, MD[b]

[a]Orthopaedic Associates of Long Island, 6 Technology Drive, Suite 100, East Setauket, New York 11733, USA
[b]DC Sportsmedicine Institute, 2021 K Street, NW, Suite 420, Washington, DC 20006, USA

Treatment of the knee that has unicompartmental osteoarthritis (OA) remains a challenging clinical problem. Despite pharmacologic advances and surgical innovations, the ideal strategy for the patient who has single-compartment degenerative disease can be complicated. Patients who are afflicted with unicompartmental disease are often younger, more active, and have higher expectations compared with their older counterparts. Furthermore, the demands imposed on their knees generally exceed those of patients who have undergone total joint arthroplasty.

The understanding and management of this problem are further confounded by the fact that so much of the data are unreliable. Most literature reflects the outcome of data generated in treating patients who have generalized OA of the knee. This information may not be extrapolated to patients who have unicompartmental OA of the knee. Given these constraints, this article outlines the current alternatives available in nonoperatively managing the symptomatic unicompartmental arthritic knee.

Significance of the problem—who are these patients?

Arthritis affects approximately 70 million Americans [1], with the cost of treatment representing 1.5% of the Gross National Product [2–4]. Nearly 50% of patients over the age of 65 years report arthritic symptoms, whereas 70% demonstrate radiographic changes [4,5]. In 1994, OA eclipsed heart disease as the leading cause of disability in the United States [6–8]. As retirement age of the baby boom generation approaches, these numbers are expected to increase dramatically.

In addition to the phenomenon of unicompartmental disease in the population, the role of arthroscopic meniscectomy in further contributing to this disease process cannot be excluded. The development of OA following even partial meniscectomy has been well established in the orthopedic literature. For example, Bolano and Grana [9] demonstrated a 50% incidence of radiographic changes 5 years following partial meniscectomy. Rangger and colleagues [10] reinforced this data, reporting arthritic changes in 38% of patients following medial meniscectomy and 24% after lateral meniscectomy. The rate of degenerative change after subtotal or complete meniscectomy is even higher, with Jorgensen and colleagues [11] demonstrating a 40% incidence

No author or institution associated with this article received anything of value as a result of their participation in the production of this manuscript, nor does any author have an affiliation with any company, product, or device named in the article.

* Corresponding author.
E-mail address: bhanypsiak@optonline.net (B.T. Hanypsiak).

of OA at 4.5 years and 89% at 14.5 years. Post-meniscectomy patients represent a significant group among patients seeking medical care for unicompartmental arthritis.

Role of lifestyle modification

Perhaps the simplest and potentially most effective measures (albeit the most difficult to implement) for nonoperatively managing the symptomatic unicompartmental arthritic knee are behavioral or lifestyle changes. Such measures should include activity modification (eliminating provocative, impact-loading stresses), weight loss (decreasing the joint reaction forces), and physical therapy (improving flexibility and strength).

The Arthritis, Diet, and Activity Promotion Trial [12] was an 18-month-long, randomized, single-blind clinical trial designed to determine the impact of long-term exercise and weight-loss (either separately or in combination) on the function, pain, and mobility in older overweight and obese adults who had knee OA. In this trial, 316 community-dwelling overweight and obese adults ages 60 years and older who had a body mass index of 28 kg/m^2 or more, knee pain, radiographic evidence of knee OA, and self-reported physical disability were randomized into healthy-lifestyle (control), diet-only, exercise-only, and diet-plus-exercise groups. The primary outcome was self-reported physical function as measured using the Western Ontario and McMaster Universities Osteoarthritis Index (WOMAC). The investigators found that the combination of modest weight loss plus moderate exercise provided better overall improvements in self-reported measures of function and pain, and in performance measures of mobility in older, overweight, and obese adults who had knee OA, compared with either intervention alone.

Orthoses

There are limited data in the literature indicating that neoprene sleeves may be effective in relieving symptoms in some patients who have knee complaints [13,14]. However, scientific evidence of their benefit is unproven, although recent data suggests some possible proprioceptive value [13]. A 2003 study in the Thai literature found small, short-term benefits in patients who had knee OA in cases where there was acute symptom exacerbation [15]. In general, these soft sleeves or braces represent no more than a treatment adjunct.

Semirigid braces could be suitable for patients who have mild to moderate unicompartmental OA. Through the three-point bending principle, unloader braces can reduce symptoms by "unloading" the affected compartment through the application of a valgus (medial compartment OA) or varus (lateral compartment OA) stress. Patients most likely to benefit from an unloader brace are those who have unicompartmental arthritis and clinically apparent pseudo-laxity on physical exam. Those patients who have fixed deformities that occur as a result of longstanding arthritis and soft tissue contracture are less likely to benefit from wearing a brace.

Several studies have demonstrated the efficacy of unloader braces in decreasing pain and improving function [13,16–19]. Potential benefits of bracing include the avoidance of surgery and its costs and complications, including protracted rehabilitation. The two major disadvantages of bracing are expense and compliance. The cost of custom bracing can be prohibitive, even for "off-the-shelf" models, a problem that is often further compounded by the refusal of many insurance programs to provide coverage. Perhaps the biggest impediment to widespread use, however, is their inconvenience, with few patients capable of complying with the demands of these braces. Fitting can be cumbersome, particularly in patients whose thighs are short and conically-shaped, and few patients can tolerate the inconvenience of use, which requires consistent compliance for maximum benefit. The true success of this alternative requires careful patient selection.

Some authors have recommended heel wedges, which theoretically decrease pressure on the knee by altering foot and ankle alignment. However, few data exist to support their effectiveness in patients who have osteoarthritic knees [20–23]. One study suggests that a lateral wedge containing an insole with a subtalar strap maintained valgus correction superior to that of lateral wedges alone. Patients who had wedges outfitted with this strap had longer clinical improvement than those who had the traditional insert [24].

Magnetic bracelets have been marketed for the treatment of arthritis pain in recent years. With the exception of a single study [25], there are few scientific data to support their efficacy.

Pharmacologic treatments

Pharmacologic treatments include oral, topical, and injectable medications. Oral medications commonly include acetaminophen, nonsteroidal anti-inflammatory drugs (NSAIDs), and recently popularized supplements.

Acetaminophen

Acetaminophen (paracetamol) has a well-established safety and efficacy profile, permitting a daily maximum dose of 4000 mg/d. According to the algorithm for the treatment of OA developed by the American College of Rheumatology, acetaminophen is the first line of therapy after nonpharmacologic modalities [26,27]. Recent literature, however, has found acetaminophen to be less efficacious. A randomized, double-blind, placebo-controlled trial of diclofenac sodium (75 mg twice daily) versus acetaminophen (1000 mg four times daily) in 82 subjects who had symptomatic OA of the medial compartment of the knee found acetaminophen to be ineffective [28].

The Ibuprofen Paracetamol Study in Osteoarthritis (IPSO) study showed that in the treatment of osteoarthritic pain, ibuprofen (400 mg/d at a single dose and 1200 mg/d at a multiple dose for 14 days) was more effective than paracetamol (either as a single dose of 1000 mg/d or a multiple dose of 3000 mg/d). Because ibuprofen and paracetamol have similar tolerability, this study indicated that the efficacy/tolerability ratio of ibuprofen is better than that of paracetamol over a 2-week period [29].

Interestingly, a placebo-controlled study was unable to demonstrate any statistically significant advantage of oral paracetamol at 4 g/d compared with placebo for the treatment of knee symptoms [30]. In the context of this finding, the advocacy of acetaminophen use in subjects who have OA of the knee should be reconsidered until evidence of its effectiveness has been determined through properly designed placebo-control studies.

Nonsteroidal anti-inflammatory drugs

Nonsteroidal anti-inflammatory drugs (NSAIDs) are usually the first line of pharmacologic treatment among orthopedists [31,32]. These medications are intended to reduce pain and inflammation associated with OA by inhibiting the production of prostaglandins in the cyclooxygenase (COX) pathway [4,33–35]. Two different COX enzymes have been described, known as COX-1 and COX-2 [34,35]. COX-1 enzymes are responsible for the production of thromboxane A_2 (platelet aggregation) and prostaglandin I_2 (gastric mucous production). COX-2 enzymes produce prostaglandin E_2, thought to be the most important inflammatory mediator.

The original NSAIDs, such as ibuprofen and naproxen sodium, nonselectively interfered with COX-1 and COX-2 enzymes [4]. They therefore successfully achieved pain relief and prevented the formation of painful inflammatory mediators, but also inhibited formation of protective prostaglandins. The non–selective adverse effects, including compromised normal gastrointestinal mucosal protection and platelet dysfunction, have been reported to be responsible for over 100,000 hospitalizations and 16,000 deaths per year [4].

The newest generation of arthritic pain medications are the COX-2 NSAIDs, including celecoxib, valdecoxib, and the recently withdrawn rofecoxib. Designed to be more selective in affecting the COX pathway, these COX-2 medications have been capable of preferentially limiting inflammation and reducing pain without interfering with the normal production of protective prostaglandins and thromboxane. In this regard, these medications have reduced the incidence of adverse effects [36]. However, despite their established efficacy, recent adverse effects, including cardiac and renal complications, have been reported [36,37] and have resulted in the voluntary withdrawal of rofecoxib. Widespread media attention has forced critical scrutiny of these drugs, including the COX-1 inhibitors. At this time, they should be prescribed with caution in patients who have established cardiovascular disease.

Another consideration influencing prescription of COX-2 inhibitors is cost, which often requires preauthorization by insurance companies and generally precludes their use in the uninsured. It is unclear at this time how recent safety issues will affect preauthorization and permission to remain on formulary for these medications.

Supplements (nutraceuticals)

Supplements have been available in one form or another for several decades. They were the first agents marketed as having the ability to relieve the symptoms of OA and to alter the disease process itself. According to the Dietary Supplement Health Education Act of 1974 (DSHEA), supplements are defined as products intended to supplement the diet that bear or contain one of the following ingredients: a vitamin, mineral, amino acid, herb, or other botanical, and are intended for ingestion as a capsule, powder, soft gel, or gel cap [38]. Supplements have experienced a meteoric rise in popularity, with sales exceeding $640 million in 2000. When combined with "functional, or healthy food," sales are forecasted to reach $21 billion in 2006 [39]. Their popularity was in part triggered by the best-selling book *The Arthritis Cure* [40], in which the authors make an impassioned but anecdotal and unscientific argument for the use of chondroitin sulfate and glucosamine sulfate in "halting, reversing and even curing osteoarthritis."

Consumer reliability is poor, partly because oral supplements are not regulated by the Food and Drug Administration (FDA) and do not fall under their guidelines for quality or efficacy. In fact, no agency holds manufacturers accountable to ensure that the contents of the container match those written on the label. Recent studies with a randomly selected group of common supplements found that a significant proportion of these products had very low or no active ingredient (N Eddington, personal communication to David Hungerford, 1997. University of Maryland School of Pharmacology. Presented at the CCJR December, 2002) [41]. Adebowale and colleagues [41] evaluated 32 products containing glucosamine or chondroitin and found that 84% failed to meet label claims. Actual concentrations of substances ranged from 0% to 115% of stated values. Similarly, *Consumer Reports* analyzed 19 products and found a wide variety of recommended dosages and a considerable range of product concentrations and label claims, some of which were not legitimate. Their report can be found in the May 2002 issue or online (available at www.consumerreports.org) [42].

Alternative therapies range from the impractical to the dangerous. Supportive data can be found extolling the virtues of almost any supplement, notwithstanding its likely unreliability. For example, randomized controlled trials of leech therapy for the treatment of knee OA have been published [43,44].

Herbal extracts have been in use for thousands of years. Because many patients are seen who already use some combination of these extracts, physicians should familiarize themselves with the most common ones and their side effects. Plant products with names like Boswellia serrata, Devil's Claw, and Chinese Thunder God are available for consumption. Obviously one must use great caution before recommending any supplement without careful consideration of its demonstrated effectiveness and certainty of its safety, especially because some of these plants are considered to be highly poisonous [45–47].

As patients increasingly turn toward supplements as a legitimate therapeutic alternative in managing their arthritis, clinicians must take their responsibility seriously in advising their patients. Recommending that patients consult available consumer data and purchase a supplement from a reputable manufacturer whose product claim has been substantiated by independent testing (such as www.consumerlab.com) is an important component of treatment.

Glucosamine and chondroitin

The literature is fairly extensive in evaluating the efficacy of chondroitin and glucosamine. Unfortunately, these data have often been biased because of industry support, precluding clear interpretation of the results.

Glucosamine sulfate is ubiquitous in the environment and is the monosaccharide precursor to glycosaminoglycans, which are the building blocks of proteoglycan, the large macromolecule that constitutes 5% to 10% of the wet weight of articular cartilage [48]. Other glycosaminoglycans include chondroitin sulfate, heparin sulfate, and dermatan sulfate. Glucosamine is extracted from shellfish such as shrimp and crab, which is an important consideration for patients who have seafood allergies [49,50]. In its sulfated form, glucosamine has a 70% absorption rate in the gastrointestinal tract with a 26% overall bioavailability. It is excreted by the kidneys and is thought to work in several ways, including (1) stimulation of chondrocyte collagen and proteoglycan production, including hyaluronic acid (HA); (2) stimulation of synoviocytes; and (3) mediation of an anti-inflammatory effect through the theorized stabilization of basement membranes and production of intracellular ground substance [50].

Chondroitin sulfate is made up of repeating disaccharide units of galactosamine sulfate and glucuronic acid, and is similar in molecular structure to heparin. Its bioavailability is variable, but is thought to be approximately 70%. Chondroitin is generally derived from cow cartilage. It works by inhibiting degradative enzymes and serving as a substrate for the production of proteoglycans [51].

Lippiello and colleagues [52] have reported a synergistic increase in proteoglycan production and a decrease in degradative enzymes in animals that were administered glucosamine and chondroitin. They also noted a protective benefit histologically in those animals administered chondroitin/glucosamine versus placebo [51]. Most studies indicate that these two products taken in combination seem to provide some level of subjective symptomatic improvement, but this benefit could take several months to appear [49]. A review of articles through the year 2000 summarized the effectiveness of clinical studies and found that overall glucosamine and chondroitin seemed to be comparable to NSAIDs without the side effects [52]. In 2000, McAlindon and colleagues [53] performed a meta-analysis of the literature through 1999, finding 17 placebo-controlled trials, 15 of which satisfied their inclusion criteria. Of these 15 trials, 13 had received some element of financial support from product manufacturers. Not surprisingly, they found that these studies exaggerated claims of clinical improvement, were flawed in design, included inadequate numbers of patients, and used nonvalidated outcome measures. In 2004, McAlindon and colleagues [54] conducted an Internet study showing again no increased effectiveness of glucosamine over placebo in treating symptoms of knee arthritis.

Subsequent to this report, several additional studies have been published regarding the efficacy of supplements. Two that are of recent interest include those of Reginster and colleagues [55] and Pavelka and colleagues [51]. In 2001, Reginster and colleagues [55] reported the results of a randomized, double-blind, placebo-controlled study of 212 patients taking either glucosamine sulfate alone or placebo over a 3-year period. They reported improvement in WOMAC scores in the glucosamine-treated cohort and a decreased incidence of radiographic changes, making this the first clinical study to suggest a possibility of a real chondroprotective benefit. In the second study, Pavelka and colleagues [51] examined the outcome of 202 patients administered glucosamine sulfate alone versus placebo who were followed subjectively and radiographically for 3 years. Like Reginster, they found better subjective scores and decreased joint-space narrowing in the glucosamine-treated group. Although there were limitations in study designs, these studies suggest a possible chondroprotective benefit and lend credence to claims that these agents can, in fact, influence the disease, not merely modify the symptoms.

Who will likely benefit from glucosamine-chondroitin therapy and how those patients can be identified remains unanswered. One study examining this question found that patients who had high type II cartilage turnover, as measured by breakdown products in the urine, were the most likely to benefit from oral supplementation [56]. Another suggested target group might consist of postmenopausal women and the elderly, the populations that are most often affected by knee OA [57,58]. In postmenopausal women, oral supplementation with glucosamine has recently been shown to increase WOMAC scores and decrease joint-space narrowing when compared with the placebo group [58].

Currently, a large multicenter study jointly sponsored by the National Institutes of Health, National Center for Complementary and Alternative Medicine, and National Institute of Arthritis and Musculoskeletal Skin Diseases is attempting to answer this question. The Glucosamine/Chondroitin Arthritis Intervention Trial is intended to test the effectiveness of these supplements in decreasing symptoms and their protective influence on articular cartilage in a large group of patients [59]. Enrollment is currently complete and final results are expected to be released in 2005.

Current dosing is weight-dependent, with the recommended daily average dose of 1500 mg glucosamine and 1200 mg chondroitin taken in combination [47,60]. However, even topical application of glucosamine and chondroitin, in association with camphor, has been shown to be somewhat effective [61].

Adverse effects include hypersensitivity in patients who are allergic to shellfish, epigastric pain, heartburn, diarrhea, drowsiness, and skin reactions [50,54]. There are no reported effects regarding blood tests, such as changes in blood count or serum chemistries [50,54]. Structural similarities of chondroitin to heparin sulfate have led to concerns about its use in patients who are anticoagulated, although no clinical adverse effects have been reported.

Similarly, there have been concerns about elevated glucose levels with the use of glucosamine in patients who are diabetic [62]. These concerns seem to have been satisfactorily addressed by a double-blind, randomized, placebo-controlled trial that failed to show a significant increase in glycosylated hemoglobin in patients who were diabetic and undergoing long-term glucosamine-chondroitin therapy [63]. One final suggested concern was the possibility of acquiring the prion-related "mad cow disease" because some chondroitin is derived from cows. However, no clinical transmissions have been reported as a consequence of chondroitin use.

Topicals

Topical medications have been commercially advertised as providing relief from the pain of arthritis. In addition to popular over-the-counter remedies such as BENGAY (Pfizer, New York, New York) and Icy Hot (Chattem, Chattanooga, Tennessee), prescription products such as lidocaine hydrochloride and topical NSAIDs have become available.

Many over-the-counter products contain capsaicin, a chemical that is thought to reversibly deplete the stores of substance P and other neurotransmitters from nerve endings [64]. An uncontrolled, open-label study of the lidocaine patch suggested good pain relief through blockade of sodium channels, a mechanism of action unique among pain relieving medications [65].

Finally, topical NSAIDs, which offer the theoretical advantage of effective local pain relief without producing harmful systemic effects, may provide the future of pain relief. A recently published, randomized, double-blind, controlled trial found topical diclofenac to be effective in the treatment of OA of the knee [66].

Injectables

Cortisone

Injectable medication has been available in the form of corticosteroids for many years, and despite the lack of high-quality scientific data supporting its use has established itself as an effective therapy for the treatment of OA [67]. By inhibiting phospholipase A_3, a membrane-associated enzyme that releases arachidonic acid from membrane lipid and initiates the COX and lipoxygenase pathways, corticosteroids transiently decrease inflammation [68,69].

Concerns about crystalline arthropathy developing as a result of frequent intra-articular corticosteroid injections have not been substantiated by randomized, controlled studies. Several trials have been published that appear to contradict this once-popular belief [69–72].

Studies that compare the symptomatic relief obtained through corticosteroid injection with that obtained through viscosupplementation have had mixed results [73,74]. No definitive conclusions can be drawn at this time.

Hyaluronic acid

HA is a repeating disaccharide unit composed of glucuronic acid and N-acetylglucosamine. It forms the backbone of aggrecan, the large macromolecule that makes up the cartilage matrix. In vivo, it is synthesized by type B synoviocytes and fibroblasts and is secreted into the joint space. Most articular HA is composed of approximately 12,500 disaccharide units whose molecular weight is 5×10^6 d. The healthy human knee contains approximately 2 mL of synovial fluid, with an HA concentration of 2.5 to 4 mg/mL [75]. HA has viscous and elastic properties that are critical to normal joint function. At low load speeds it acts as a lubricant, and at faster movements as a shock absorber [75,76]. In OA, the concentration of HA is reduced by one half to one third of normal. The molecular size of HA is also reduced [76,77]. This combination leads to decreased effec-

tiveness and increased wear rates, and is the basis for clinical strategies through viscosupplementation.

Several injectable variations of HA have been introduced. Because the FDA permitted approval as a "device" rather than a medication, HA was not required to meet the stringent criteria by the FDA for efficacy demanded of drugs in clinical trials [76].

The various commercially available preparations of HA are all derived from the fractionated hyalurons from rooster combs. HA is thought to lack antigenicity and, once absorbed, is metabolized by the liver. Several mechanisms of action for HA have been suggested, including anti-inflammatory effects, anabolic effects, analgesic effects, chondroprotective effects, and improved viscoelasticity [76,77].

Although the exact mechanism of action remains unknown, HA is unlikely to achieve any beneficial effect based on lubrication because any mechanical contribution is ephemeral. Animal studies have shown a rapid clearance of HA from the joint [77,78], and it is estimated that HA is completely absorbed from the joint within hours to days of its administration in humans. Radiolabeling studies show that HA is absorbed by the synovium within 2 hours and by cartilage within 6 hours. In sheep, its mean half-life in normal joints is 20.8 hours and in the acutely inflamed knee only 11.5 hours [77,78].

Despite the rapid metabolism and clearance from the joint, clinical studies show improvement that far outlasts the duration of the injectable HA itself. Such evidence underscores the fact that HA does not exert its predominant clinical effect through viscosupplementation, or simply replacing degraded HA.

Commercial forms vary in their specific composition with respect to the concentration of the HA and the actual molecular form. Formaldehyde has been used to cross-link, and thereby increase, the molecular weight (hylan G-F 20; Genzyme, Cambridge, Massachusetts) in an attempt to more accurately replicate the normal HA molecule. Despite such efforts, few data exist to prove the superiority of large over small molecular weight HA, with the exception of work by a single author [79]. Furthermore, the formaldehyde used in cross-linking has been associated with a small incidence of adverse reactions after injection [75,79].

Animal and human studies have shown a positive overall benefit to the use of HA in treating mild to moderate OA [80–85]. Animal models have shown some evidence of a chondroprotective benefit. A summary of the clinical literature and a meta-analysis of randomized controlled trials have recently been published in the *Journal of the American Academy of Orthopaedic Surgery* [76] and *Journal of Bone and*

Joint Surgery: American Volume respectively [85]. These studies confirmed the safety and efficacy of HA injections and generally demonstrated subjective improvement when compared with placebo control at 6 months. No conclusions, however, could be drawn regarding efficacy of high versus low molecular weight products [85].

Few adverse reactions have been reported (approximately 1%) with HA injections, and those that have occurred have been mild with increased pain, warmth, or swelling at the injection site [76]. More severe reactions have been described and are known as pseudo-septic reactions for their resemblance to the infected knee [85,86]. One series reported a 27% incidence of these clinically significant inflammatory reactions [80]. This incidence was attributed to the formaldehyde used in cross-linking the Synvisc preparation.

The injection series can be repeated without any apparent limit, with one study showing improvement after each round [87]. However, a second study demonstrated an increased rate of local reaction with each subsequent series of injections [88]. Although a second course of viscosupplementation has been shown to be safe and effective [89], the incidence of inflammatory reaction has been shown to increase with subsequent therapeutic rounds of injections and is nearly always associated with the use of cross-linked sodium hyaluronates [90].

Pricing is variable depending on the product used, the number of injections required, and the insurance company. Preauthorization is often required for insurance purposes. A recent publication found appropriately indicated treatment with Synvisc to be no more costly than other conventional treatments [91].

In summary, HA may be a reasonable alternative for some patients who have painful OA, especially those who are intolerant of other medications or who have failed other nonoperative treatment. It can be useful in conjunction with other treatments, with some physicians using it in combination with corticosteroid injections—an "off label" use [92].

Arthroscopy

Arthroscopy has long been considered an effective alternative in the treatment of OA [93–103]. However, a recent study by Moseley and colleagues [102] in the *New England Journal of Medicine* called its value into question. In a randomized, double-blind study of 165 Veterans Affairs patients who had OA, the investigators found no difference in outcome in groups treated with lavage, debridement, or sham

surgery. Their conclusion was that arthroscopy was an "expensive and unnecessary" modality in the treatment of knee OA.

Many authors have since correctly pointed out the limitations of this study, including flawed inclusion and exclusion criteria, insufficient power analysis, and use of nonvalidated outcome measures. The investigators failed to provide important information such as body weight, knee alignment, instability, and the presence or absence of knee effusion. Patients who had mechanical symptoms (eg, those most likely to benefit from surgery) were specifically excluded. These criticisms notwithstanding, the study was significant in emphasizing the value of nonoperative treatment and reinforcing that patients who have arthritis but no mechanical symptoms might not be prognostically good arthroscopic candidates.

This study also highlights the inadequacy of the current scientific database in treating this condition. Well-designed, prospective, double-blind studies are currently underway in hopes that they will convincingly demonstrate the efficacy of arthroscopy in an appropriately indicated group of patients who have OA. Clinical variables in the decision-making process should include the presence of mechanical symptoms, alignment, body mass, the presence of effusions, activity level, and patient demands. All of these require careful clinical consideration. Prognostic factors influencing outcome in these patients have been recently reviewed by Hunt and colleagues [103] in the *Journal of the American Academy of Orthopaedic Surgery.*

Summary

Management of the unicompartmental osteoarthritic knee is challenging. Recent treatment modalities, including NSAIDs, supplements, and injectable HA, have provided clinically effective adjuncts. Supplements seem to be most effective in treating mild to moderate OA. Wide product variability mandates familiarization by health care providers. The widely advertised chondroprotective benefit has not been convincingly proven and awaits further outcome studies. HA seems to be clinically effective in patients who have mild to moderate OA, and has a low complication rate. Its effectiveness, however, is probably not achieved through its marketed viscosupplementation mechanism. Further research will allow a better determination of its exact position in the OA management algorithm. In the future, treatment of OA will most likely focus on prevention, and biologic manipulation such as gene therapy may eventually render even today's "advanced" therapeutic alternatives obsolete.

References

[1] Arthritis Foundation. Available at: www.arthritis.org.
[2] Simon LS. Viscosupplementation therapy with intraarticular hyaluronic acid. Osteoarthritis 1999;25: 345–57.
[3] Cefalu CA, Waddell DS. Viscosupplementation: treatment alternative for osteoarthritis of the knee. Geriatrics 1999;54:51–7.
[4] Bert JM, Gasser SI. Approach to the osteoarthritic knee in the aging athlete: debridement to osteotomy. Arthroscopy 2002;18:107–10.
[5] Lane NE, Thompson JM. Management of osteoarthritis in the primary care setting: an evidence-based approach to treatment. Am J Med 1997;103: 25S–30S.
[6] Guccione AA, Felson DT, Anderson JJ, et al. The effects of specific medical conditions on the functional limitations of elders in the Framingham Study. Am J Public Health 1994;84:351–8.
[7] Altman RD, Moskowitz R. Intraarticular sodium hyaluronate (Hyalgan) in the treatment of patients with osteoarthritis of the knee: a randomized clinical trial. J Rheumatol 1998;25:2203–12.
[8] Owings MF, Kozak LJ. Ambulatory and inpatient procedures in the United States, 1996. Vital and health statistics. Series 13. No 139. Hyattsville (MD): National Center for Health Statistics; 1998 [DHHS publication no. (PHS) 99–1710].
[9] Bolano LE, Grana WA. Isolated arthroscopic partial meniscectomy. Functional radiographic evaluation at five years. Am J Sports Med 1993;21:432–7.
[10] Rangger C, Klestil T, Gloetzer W, et al. Osteoarthritis after arthroscopic partial meniscectomy. Am J Sports Med 1995;23:240–4.
[11] Jorgensen U, Sonne-Holm S, Lauridsen F, et al. Long-term follow-up of meniscectomy in athletes: a prospective longitudinal study. J Bone Joint Surg Br 1987;69:80–3.
[12] Messier SP, Loeser RF, Miller GD, et al. Exercise and dietary weight loss in overweight and obese older adults with knee osteoarthritis: the Arthritis, Diet, and Activity Promotion Trial. Arthritis Rheum 2004; 50(5):1501–10.
[13] Kirkley A, Webster-Bogaert S, Litchfield R, et al. The effect of bracing on varus gonarthrosis. J Bone Joint Surg Am 1999;81:539–48.
[14] Brouwer R, Jakma T, Verhagen A, et al. Braces and orthoses for treating osteoarthritis of the knee. Cochrane Database Syst Rev 2005;1:CD004020.
[15] Pajareya K, Chadchavalpanichaya N, Timdang S. Effectiveness of an elastic knee sleeve for patients with knee osteoarthritis: a randomized single-blinded controlled trial. J Med Assoc Thai 2003;86(6):535–42.

[16] Horlick S, Loomer R. Valgus knee bracing for medial gonarthrosis. Clin J Sport Med 1993;3:251–5.
[17] Lindenfeld T, Hewett T, Andriacchi T. Joint loading with valgus bracing in patients with varus gonarthrosis. Clin Orthop 1997;344:290–7.
[18] Finger S, Paulos L. Clinical and biomechanical evaluation of the unloading brace. J Knee Surg 2002;15: 155–9.
[19] Self BP, Greenwald RM, Pflaster DS. A biomechanical analysis of a medial unloading brace for osteoarthritis in the knee. Arthritis Care Res 2000;13(4): 191–7.
[20] Tohyama H, Yasuda K, Kaneda K. Treatment of osteoarthritis of the knee with heel wedges. Int Orthop 1991;15:31–3.
[21] Wolfe SA, Brueckmann FR. Conservative treatment of genu valgus and varum with medial/lateral heel wedges. Indiana Med 1991;84:614–5.
[22] Keating EM, Faris PM, Ritter MA, et al. Use of lateral heel and sole wedges in the treatment of medial osteoarthritis of the knee. Orthop Rev 1993;22: 921–4.
[23] Pham T, Maillefert JF, Hudry C, et al. Laterally elevated wedged insoles in the treatment of medial knee osteoarthritis. A two-year prospective randomized controlled study. Osteoarthritis Cartilage 2004; 12(1):46–55.
[24] Toda Y, Tsukimura N. A six-month follow-up of a randomized trial comparing the efficacy of a lateral-wedge insole with subtalar strapping and an in-shoe lateral-wedge insole in patients with varus deformity osteoarthritis of the knee. Arthritis Rheum 2004; 50(10):3129–36.
[25] Harlow T, Greaves C, White A, et al. Randomised controlled trial of magnetic bracelets for relieving pain in osteoarthritis of the hip and knee. BMJ 2004;329(7480):1450–4.
[26] Hochberg MC, Altman RD, Brandt KD, et al. Guidelines for the medical management of osteoarthritis. Parts I and II. Osteoarthritis of the hip and knee. Arthritis Rheum 1995;38:1535–46.
[27] Hochberg MC, Dougados M. Pharmacological therapy of osteoarthritis. Best Pract Res Clin Rheumatol 2001;15:583–93.
[28] Case JP, Baliunas AJ, Block JA. Lack of efficacy of acetaminophen in treating symptomatic knee osteoarthritis: a randomized, double-blind, placebo-controlled comparison trial with diclofenac sodium. Arch Intern Med 2003;163(2):169–78.
[29] Boureau F, Schneid H, Zeghari N, et al. The IPSO study: ibuprofen, paracetamol study in osteoarthritis. A randomised comparative clinical study comparing the efficacy and safety of ibuprofen and paracetamol analgesic treatment of osteoarthritis of the knee or hip. Ann Rheum Dis 2004;63(9):1028–34.
[30] Miceli-Richard C, Le Bars M, Schmidely N, et al. Paracetamol in osteoarthritis of the knee. Ann Rheum Dis 2004;63(8):923–30.
[31] Goorman SD, Watanabe TK, Miller EH, et al.

Functional outcome in knee osteoarthritis after treatment with Hylan G-F 20: a prospective study. Arch Phys Med Rehabil 2000;81:479–83.

[32] Cole BJ, Harner CD. Degenerative arthritis of the knee in active patients: evaluation and management. J Am Acad Orthop Surg 1999;7:389–402.

[33] Stanley KL, Weaver JE. Pharmacologic management of pain and inflammation in athletes. Clin Sports Med 1998;17:375–92.

[34] Dray A, Urban L. New pharmacological strategies for pain relief. Annu Rev Pharmacol Toxicol 1996;36:253–80.

[35] Polisson R. NSAIDs: practical and therapeutic considerations in their selection. Am J Med 1996;100:315–65.

[36] Solomon G. The use of cox-2-specific inhibitors with specific attention to use in patients requiring orthopedic surgical interventions. Orthopedic Special Edition 2002;8:11–3.

[37] Nelson C. Pondering Vioxx: easier on stomach, harder on heart? Sports Med Digest 2001;23:40–3.

[38] U.S. Food and Drug Administration Center for Food Safety and Applied Nutrition. Dietary Supplement Health and Education Act of 1994. Available at: http://vm.cfsan.fda.gov/~dms/dietsupp.html. Accessed December 1, 1995.

[39] Packaged Facts, NY, NY. The US market for nutraceuticals. Available at: www.packagedfacts.com/pub/186556.html#pagetop. Accessed September 1, 2000.

[40] Theodosakis J, Adderly B, Fox B. The arthritis cure. New York: St. Martin's Press; 1997.

[41] Adebowale AO, Cox DS, Liang Z, et al. Analysis of glucosamine and chondroitin sulfate content in marketed products and the Caco-2 permeability of chondroitin sulfate raw materials. J Am Nutraceutical Assoc 2000;3:37–44.

[42] Horstman J. The Arthritis Foundation's guide to alternative therapies. Atlanta (GA): The Arthritis Foundation; 1999.

[43] Michalsen A, Klotz S, Ludtke R, et al. Effectiveness of leech therapy in osteoarthritis of the knee: a randomized controlled trial. Ann Intern Med 2003;139(9):724–30.

[44] Michalsen A, Moebus S, Spahn G, et al. Leech therapy for symptomatic treatment of knee osteoarthritis: results and implications of a pilot study. Altern Ther Health Med 2002;8(5):84–8.

[45] Wegener T, Lupke NP. Treatment of patients with arthrosis of hip or knee with an aqueous extract of devil's claw (Harpagophytum procumbens DC). Phytother Res 2003;17(10):1165–72.

[46] Halpern B. The knee crisis handbook. Rodale: New York; 2003.

[47] Kimmatkar N, Thawani V, Hingorani L, et al. Efficacy and tolerability of Boswellia serrata extract in treatment of osteoarthritis of knee–a randomized double blind placebo controlled trial. Phytomedicine 2003;10(1):3–7.

[48] Brief AA, Maurer SG, Di Cesare PE. Use of glucosamine and chondroitin sulfate in the management of osteoarthritis. J Am Acad Orthop Surg 2001;9:71–7.

[49] Doulens KM, Joshi AB, Lichtman DM. Glucosamine and chondroitin in the treatment of osteoarthritis. Womens Health 2003;6:27–32.

[50] Shmerling R, Ulbricht C, Basch E. Options for arthritis pain. Newsweek December 2, 2002:53.

[51] Pavelka K, Gatterova J, Olejarova M, et al. Glucosamine sulfate use and delay of progression of knee osteoarthritis. Arch Intern Med 2002;162:2113–23.

[52] Lippiello L, Woodward J, Karpman R, et al. In vivo chondroprotection and metabolic synergy of glucosamine and chondroitin sulfate. Clin Orthop 2000;381:229–40.

[53] McAlindon TE, LaValley MP, Gulin JP, et al. Glucosamine and chondroitin for treatment of osteoarthritis. JAMA 2000;283:1469–75.

[54] McAlindon T, Formica M, LaValley M, et al. Effectiveness of glucosamine for symptoms of knee osteoarthritis: results from an internet-based randomized double-blind controlled trial. Am J Med 2004;117(9):643–9.

[55] Reginster JY, Deroisy R, Rovati LC, et al. Long term effects of glucosamine sulphate on osteoarthritis progression: A randomised, placebo-controlled clinical trial. Lancet 2001;357:251–6.

[56] Christgau S, Henrotin Y, Tanko LB, et al. Osteoarthritic patients with high cartilage turnover show increased responsiveness to the cartilage protecting effects of glucosamine sulphate. Clin Exp Rheumatol 2004;22(1):36–42.

[57] Gokhale JA, Frenkel SR, Dicesare PE. Estrogen and osteoarthritis. Am J Orthopedics 2004;33:71–80.

[58] Bruyere O, Pavelka K, Rovati LC, et al. Glucosamine sulfate reduces osteoarthritis progression in postmenopausal women with knee osteoarthritis: evidence from two 3-year studies. Menopause 2004;11(2):138–43.

[59] Biggee BA, McAlindon TE. Glucosamine for osteoarthritis: part I, review of clinical evidence. Med Health R I 2004;87(6):176–9.

[60] Leffler CT, Philippi AF, Leffler SG, et al. Glucosamine, chondroitin, and manganese ascorbate for degenerative joint disease of the knee or low back: a randomized, double-blind, placebo-controlled pilot study. Mil Med 1999;164:85–91.

[61] Cohen M, Wolfe R, Mai T, et al. A randomized, double blind, placebo controlled trial of a topical cream containing glucosamine sulfate, chondroitin sulfate, and camphor for osteoarthritis of the knee. J Rheumatol 2003;30(3):523–8.

[62] Adams ME. Hype about glucosamine. Lancet 1999;354:353–4.

[63] Scroggie DA, Albright A, Harris MD. The effect of glucosamine-chondroitin supplementation on glycosylated hemoglobin levels in patients with type 2 diabetes mellitus: a placebo-controlled, double-blinded, randomized clinical trial. Arch Intern Med 2003;163(13):1587–90.

[64] Rains C, Bryson HM. Topical capsaicin. A review of its pharmacological properties and therapeutic potential in post-herpetic neuralgia, diabetic neuropathy and osteoarthritis. Drugs Aging 1995;7(4):317–28.

[65] Galer BS, Sheldon E, Patel N, et al. Topical lidocaine patch 5% may target a novel underlying pain mechanism in osteoarthritis. Curr Med Res Opin 2004; 20(9):1455–8.

[66] Roth SH, Shainhouse JZ. Efficacy and safety of a topical diclofenac solution (Pennsaid, Dimethaid Research Incorporated, Markham, Ontario, Canada) in the treatment of primary osteoarthritis of the knee: a randomized, double blind, vehicle-controlled clinical trial. Arch Intern Med 2004;164(18):2017–23.

[67] Fadale P, Wiggins M. Corticosteroid injections: their use and abuse. J Am Acad Orthop Surg 1994; 2:133–40.

[68] Noerdlinger M, Fadale P. The role of injectable corticosteroids in orthopedics. Orthopedics 2001; 24:400–5.

[69] Raynauld JP, Buckland-Wright C, Ward R, et al. Safety and efficacy of long-term intraarticular steroid injections in osteoarthritis of the knee: a randomized, double-blind, placebo-controlled trial. Arthritis Rheum 2003;48(2):370–7.

[70] Cole BJ, Schumacher HR. Injectable corticosteroids in modern practice. J Am Acad Orthop Surg 2005;13: 37–46.

[71] Roberts WN, Babcock EA, Breitbach SA, et al. Corticosteroid injection in rheumatoid arthritis does not increase rate of total joint arthroplasty. J Rheumatol 1996;23:1001–4.

[72] Huppertz HI, Tschammler A, Horwitz AE, et al. Intraarticular corticosteroids for chronic arthritis in children: efficacy and effects on cartilage and growth. J Pediatr 1995;127:317–21.

[73] Caborn D, Rush J, Lanzer W, et al. Synvisc 901 Study Group. A randomized, single-blind comparison of the efficacy and tolerability of hylan G-F 20 and triamcinolone hexacetonide in patients with osteoarthritis of the knee. J Rheumatol 2004;31(2): 333–43.

[74] Leopold SS, Redd BB, Warme WJ, et al. Corticosteroid compared with hyaluronic acid injections for the treatment of osteoarthritis of the knee. A prospective, randomized trial. J Bone Joint Surg Am 2003;85A(7):1197–203.

[75] Simon LS. Viscosupplementation therapy with intra-articular hyaluronic acid. Osteoarthritis 1999;25: 345–57.

[76] Watterson JR, Esdaile J. Viscosupplementation: therapeutic mechanisms and clinical potential in osteoarthritis of the knee. J Am Acad Orthop Surg 2000; 8:277–84.

[77] Marshall KW, Manolopoulos V, Mercer K, et al. Amelioration of disease severity by intraarticular hylan therapy in bilateral canine osteoarthritis. J Orthop Res 2000;18:416–25.

[78] Fraser JRE, Kimpton WG, Pierscionek BK, et al.

[79] The kinetics of hyaluronan in normal and acutely inflamed synovial joints: observations with experimental arthritis in sheep. Semin Arthritis Rheum 1993;22:9–17.

[79] Wobig M, Bach G, Beks P, et al. The role of elastoviscosity in the efficacy of viscosupplementation for osteoarthritis of the knee: a comparison of hylan GF-20 and a lower-molecular-weight hyaluronan. Clin Ther 1999;21:1549–62.

[80] Puttick MPE, Wade JP, Chalmers A, et al. Acute local reactions after intraarticular hylan for osteoarthritis of the knee. J Rheumatol 1995;22:1311–4.

[81] Adams ME. An analysis of clinical studies of the use of crosslinked hyaluronan, hylan, in the treatment of osteoarthritis. J Rheumatol 1993;20:16–8.

[82] Scale D, Wobig M, Wolpert W. Viscosupplementation of osteoarthritic knees with hylan: a treatment schedule study. Curr Ther Res 1994;55:220–32.

[83] Adams ME, Atkinson MH, Lussier AJ, et al. The role of viscosupplementation with hylan g-f 20 (Synvisc) in the treatment of osteoarthritis of the knee: a Canadian multicenter trial comparing hylan g-f 20 alone, hylan g-f 20 with non-steroidal anti-inflammatory drugs (NSAIDs) and NSAIDs alone. Osteoarthritis Cartilage 1995;3:213–26.

[84] Yoshioka M, Shimizu C, Harwood F, et al. The effects of hyaluronan during the development of osteoarthritis. Osteoarthritis Cartilage 1997;5:251–60.

[85] Wang C, Lin J, Chang C, et al. Therapeutic effects of hyaluronic acid on osteoarthritis of the knee: a meta-analysis of randomized controlled trials. J Bone Joint Surg Am 2004;86(3):538–45.

[86] Kelly MA, Kurzweil PR, Moskowitz RW. Intraarticular hyaluronans in knee osteoarthritis: rationale and practical considerations. Am J Ortho 2004; 33(Suppl 2):15–22.

[87] Kotz R, Kolarz G. Intra-articular hyaluronic acid: duration of effect and results of repeated treatment cycles. Am J Orthop 1999;28:5–7.

[88] Leopold SS, Warme WJ, Pettis PD, et al. Increased frequency of acute local reaction to intra-articular hylan GF-20 (Synvisc) in patients receiving more than one course of treatment. J Bone Joint Surg Am 2002;84:1619–23.

[89] Waddell DD, Cefalu CA, Bricker DC. An open-label study of a second course of hylan G-F 20 for the treatment of pain associated with knee osteoarthritis. Curr Med Res Opin 2003;19(6):499–507.

[90] Goldberg VM, Coutts RD. Pseudoseptic reactions to hylan viscosupplementation. Clin Orthop 2004; 419:130–7.

[91] Kahan A, Lleu PL, Salin L. Prospective randomized study comparing the medicoeconomic benefits of Hylan GF-20 vs. conventional treatment in knee osteoarthritis. Joint Bone Spine 2003;70(4):276–81.

[92] Coutts RD, Waddell DD. Viscosupplementaion for osteoarthritis of the knee. Orthopedics 2004;27(5): 470–1.

[93] Kalunian KC, Moreland LW, Klashman DJ, et al.

Visually-guided irrigation in patients with early knee osteoarthritis: A multicenter randomized, controlled trial. Osteoarthritis Cartilage 2000;8:412–8.

[94] Baumgaertner MR, Cannon Jr WD, Vittore JM, et al. Arthroscopic debridement of the arthritic knee. Clin Orthop 1990;253:197–202.

[95] Bert JM, Maschka K. The arthroscopic treatment of unicompartmental gonarthrosis: A five-year follow-up study of abrasion arthroplasty plus arthroscopic debridement and arthroscopic debridement alone. Arthroscopy 1989;5:25–32.

[96] Chang RW, Falconer J, Stulberg SD, et al. A randomized, controlled trial of arthroscopic surgery versus closed-needle joint lavage for patients with osteoarthritis of the knee. Arthritis Rheum 1993; 36:289–96.

[97] Livesley PJ, Doherty M, Needhoff M, et al. Arthroscopic lavage of osteoarthritic knees. J Bone Joint Surg Br 1991;73:922–6.

[98] Sprague III NF. Arthroscopic debridement for degenerative knee joint disease. Clin Orthop 1981;160: 118–23.

[99] Salisbury RB, Nottage WM, Gardner V. The effect of alignment on results in arthroscopic debridement of the degenerative knee. Clin Orthop 1985;198: 268–72.

[100] Richards Jr RN, Lonergan RP. Arthroscopic surgery for relief of pain in the osteoarthritic knee. Orthopedics 1984;7:1705–7.

[101] McLaren AC, Blokker CP, Fowler PJ, et al. Arthroscopic debridement of the knee for osteoarthritis. Can J Surg 1991;34:595–8.

[102] Moseley JB, O'Malley K, Petersen NJ, et al. A controlled trial of arthroscopic surgery for osteoarthritis of the knee. N Engl J Med 2002;347:81–8.

[103] Hunt SA, Jazrawi LM, Sherman OH. Arthroscopic management of osteoarthritis of the knee. J Am Acad Orthop Surg 2002;10:356–63.

ELSEVIER
SAUNDERS

Orthop Clin N Am 36 (2005) 413–417

ORTHOPEDIC
CLINICS
OF NORTH AMERICA

The Indications for Arthroscopic Debridement for Osteoarthritis of the Knee

Brian Day, MD

University of British Columbia, Department of Orthopaedics, 2836 Ash Street, Vancouver, British Columbia V5Z 3C6, Canada

What is arthroscopic debridement?

The term *arthroscopic debridement* as described for the treatment of osteoarthritis of the knee has never been clearly defined. Although the literature on this topic is vast, the lack of clear descriptions and definitions of the specific pathology being treated, the failure to specify or standardize the procedure being performed, and the lack of consensus on indications and efficacy have led to some unscientific and at times irrational debate on its role.

Most would agree that the term arthroscopic debridement would include lavage and the removal of loose bodies, debris, mobile fragments of articular cartilage, unstable torn menisci, and impinging osteophytes. However, it is clear from the literature that drilling, abrasion chondroplasty, microfracture, saucerization, notchplasty, osteophyte removal, synovectomy, and arthrolysis are also performed simultaneously in many clinical series. This lack of standardization is illustrated most clearly in the example where Moseley and colleagues [1] believe that the term *lavage* includes meniscectomy.

Evolution of arthroscopic debridement

The use of joint lavage for arthritis dates back to Bircher [2] in 1922 and Burman and colleagues [3] in 1934. Burman performed arthroscopy in two patients and reported great symptomatic relief, presumably because of the lavage. In recent years, several

E-mail address: bday@telus.net

authors studied the role of arthroscopic lavage and found that, although it may result in improved symptoms, the benefits are often short-lasting. In a randomized, single-blinded prospective trial comparing medical management with knee irrigation, a statistically significant improvement in pain and function was found in the irrigation group [4]. In another study, lavage with physiotherapy was shown to be superior to physiotherapy alone. The improvement was still evident 1 year later [5]. Others have failed to demonstrate any statistically significant benefit from lavage [6].

Magnuson [7] reported on the role of open debridement of the knee joint. He performed an open arthrotomy and removal of synovium, osteophytes, and damaged or diseased cartilage. Based on the fact that articular cartilage did not regenerate well, Pridie [8] proposed drilling of exposed subchondral bone with the aim of stimulating a fibrocartilaginous repair. The theory was that this tissue may provide some functional capacity. In 1959, he reported a success rate of 65% in his patients. Arthroscopic procedures such as abrasion arthroplasty and microfracture later evolved and were based on similar biologic theories.

Staging and classification of the severity of osteoarthritis have never been standardized in the literature. The simple scale outlined by Jackson and Dieterichs [9] uses clinical and arthroscopic criteria and includes a radiologic factor in its grading. Many retain the standard Outerbridge classification for chondral lesions, although it was designed for the classification of "chondromalacia" [10].

The controversial Wren–Moseley [1] study gained publicity and notoriety, much of it in the lay press. In this study, inclusion and exclusion criteria were ill defined and data collection was inadequate. Chambers and colleagues [11] provided an authoritative scientific rebuttal of the study, concluding that methodology problems with the study design invalidated Moseley et al's results. Data interpretation was based on false premises and there was inadequate documentation and classification. Poor statistical methods and a self-produced, nonvalidated measurement tool were used. In applying the standard power formula for equivalence studies to their data, all were between 14% to 70% and below the conventional power level of 80% needed to show equivalence.

The single surgeon's (Moseley) technique was not described and could not be compared with any known standard. Mechanical symptoms were not considered, and the presence of knee effusions not documented. Body weight and radiology assessment and scale were poorly described, and knee alignment and instability were not documented. The sham surgical procedure did not fit the required criteria or definition (inert and innocuous) of a placebo. Lavage was one of the study comparables, but meniscectomy was included as a component of knee lavage. Contrary to claims, there were two previously controlled randomized studies that confirmed the efficacy of arthroscopic debridement in properly selected patients. Hubbard [12], in a prospective randomized trial involving 76 knees, found that at 1 year, 80% of the debridement group and 14% of the washout group were pain-free, and at 5 years, 59% of the debridement 12% of the washout group remained pain-free. Merchan and Galindo [13] performed a randomized clinical trial involving 80 patients who had mean 24 months follow-up. The investigators excluded patients who had an angular deformity greater than 15°. One group underwent arthroscopic debridement and controls were treated nonoperatively with nonsteroidal anti-inflammatory drugs and activity modification. Seventy-five percent of the arthroscopically

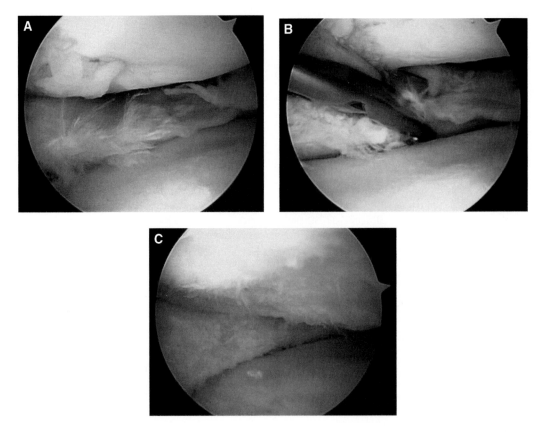

Fig. 1. (*A*) Medial compartment of left knee in a 59-year-old man who has osteoarthritis. (*B*) Arthroscopic debridement with removal of unstable meniscus and articular cartilage. (*C*) Postarthroscopic appearance.

treated patients improved, compared with only 16% of the nonoperative group. There have also been long-term follow-up studies on the value of arthroscopic debridement for osteoarthritis. Fond and colleagues [14] studied 36 patients after knee arthroscopy for arthritic symptoms refractory to conservative treatment. The procedure involved debridement of meniscal lesions, stabilization of chondral defects, removal of impinging osteophytes, and notchplasty. At 5 years, 25 of the 36 patients were satisfied with good to excellent results. The reduction in pain is probably caused by many factors, including the washout effects of lavage, reduced impingement, and improved range of motion and joint mechanics that result from reduction in friction between the opposing articular surfaces. Fig. 1 illustrates the pre- and postarthroscopic debridement appearances in the medial compartment of the knee of a 59-year-old man. Bonamo and Kessler [15] studied prognostic factors for patients older than 40 years undergoing arthroscopic partial meniscectomy and debridement of coexisting articular cartilage damage. The control group did not have clinically significant articular degeneration. Of 181 who completed the study, 63 were in Outerbridge classification I and II and 118 were in the more severe categories III and IV. The investigators showed that patients who had more severe arthritis were less satisfied with their results.

Patient selection for arthroscopic debridement

Determining which patients are suitable for arthroscopic debridement should be based on a detailed clinical evaluation. The current literature suggests that patients who have a short history and a sudden onset of mechanical symptoms and also have knee effusions are likely to do best. Meniscal symptoms and signs; synovitis or synovial impingement; osteophytic impingement; and catching or locking caused by loose bodies favor a good outcome. Significant instability or malalignment are poor prognostic factors. Patients who have radiographic signs of advanced degeneration are unlikely to benefit. Radiographs should include standing anteroposterior and 45° flexion weight-bearing posteroanterior views, and lateral and patellofemoral views. In some patients, such as those who may be candidates for osteotomy or arthroplasty, long-standing films to measure the anatomic and mechanical axes are needed. Complete loss of joint space, polycompartment disease, or major malalignment make a successful outcome from arthroscopic debridement less likely. Maintenance of

some joint space, the presence of loose bodies amenable to removal, and chondrocalcinosis are positive prognostic factors.

Arthroscopic meniscectomy in severe arthritis

Pearse and Craig [16] showed that arthroscopic partial meniscectomy, even in the presence of Outerbridge grade IV degenerative changes, will improve symptoms in many patients who have symptomatic meniscal tears, and that the benefit may last many years (Fig. 2). The removal of torn menisci did not increase the progression of the osteoarthritis. The ability to delay or avoid more major surgical interventions, with their increased morbidity, is clearly of great benefit. The investigators disproved the claims of others [17] who had suggested that partial meniscectomy in a severely arthritic joint may accelerate the progression of osteoarthritis and precipitate the need for joint replacement.

Arthroscopy and the stiff arthritic knee

Puddu and colleagues [18] showed the value of arthroscopic removal of the anterior tibial osteophyte in the treatment of flexion deformity of the knee in patients undergoing arthroscopic debridement for osteoarthritis of the knee. This procedure may be particularly valuable and was found to be effective in relieving pain in such patients. Fond and colleagues

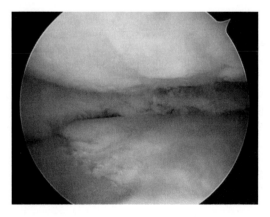

Fig. 2. Symptomatic medial meniscus tear with grade 4 tibial plateau changes.

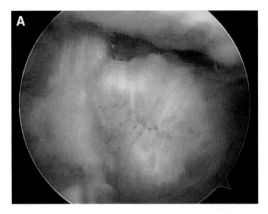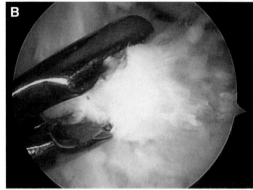

Fig. 3. (*A*) Anterior impinging osteophyte limiting extension. (*B*) Removal of impinging osteophytes.

[14] had also found that arthroscopic debridement and osteophytic removal was beneficial, but emphasized that the best results were obtained with a flexion deformity that was less than 10°. Fig. 3 illustrates the type of anteriorly impinging osteophyte that would limit extension. The removal of such a lesion will eventually lead to improved range of motion and reduced pain.

Role of arthroscopy as an adjunct to open surgery

Presurgical arthroscopic debridement may be needed in patients undergoing realignment procedures. Arthroscopic debridement combined with unloader bracing may allow one to delay or avoid osteotomy. It is clear that osteotomy is more likely to succeed if loose bodies, impinging chondral fragments, and unstable meniscal tears are dealt with at the same time. Arthroscopic investigation of post-osteotomy pain or failed osteotomies is sometimes able to prevent or delay the need for knee arthroplasty. Several authors, including Boldin and colleagues [20], have shown that arthroscopic debridement in patients who have total knee arthroplasties is valuable in the diagnosis and treatment of postoperative dysfunction, such as arthrofibrosis, soft tissue impingement, patella instability, infection, breakdown of implants, and hemarthrosis. Clear imaging of post-arthroplasty problems is difficult and arthroscopic examination and debridement may help in the management of these difficult problems.

Arthroscopic debridement is also a component of many other procedures, such as autologous chondrocyte procedures, osteochondral grafts, Uni-Spacer (Zimmer Inc, Warsaw, IN) insertion, meniscal transplantation, and anterior and posterior ligament reconstruction.

Summary

As with almost all surgical treatments in orthopedics, most of the published literature has comprised retrospective studies. Most authors report improvement in 50% to 80% of patients; however, as one would expect with a degenerative condition, results deteriorate with time. The evidence supporting the therapeutic value of arthroscopic debridement of the knee is overwhelming [9,12–16,18,19,21–24]. However, there is a need for better-designed clinical trials comparing arthroscopic debridement to established alternative treatments. Despite the claims of some nonphysician ethicists, the author does not consider so-called placebo or "sham" surgery to be ethical. The Moseley study illustrates that a prospective, randomized, controlled study is unreliable if invalid statistical methods are used or when clinical documentation of important variables is ignored. The most important factor in determining success is proper patient selection, and many who have osteoarthritis of the knee will not benefit from arthroscopic debridement. Patients who have end-stage osteoarthritis or severe malalignment and those who do not have mechanical symptoms are unlikely to improve. The important considerations are how effective the treatment is and whether the expected benefits justify the risks, potential complications, and cost [25]. An objective analysis of outcome studies in patients who have osteoarthritis of the knee joint clearly shows that properly selected patients will benefit greatly from arthroscopic debridement and many will be saved from the increased morbidity and potential complications of alternative treatments.

References

[1] Moseley JB, O'Malley K, Petersen NJ, et al. A controlled trial of arthroscopic surgery for osteoarthritis of the knee. N Engl J Med 2002;347:81–8.

[2] Bircher E. Beitrag zur pathologie (arthritis deformans) und diagnose der meniscus-verletzungen (arthroendoskopie). Beitr Klin Chir 1922;127:239–50.

[3] Burman MS, Finkelstein H, Mayer L. Arthroscopy of the knee joint. J Bone Joint Surg 1934;16:255–68.

[4] Ike RW, Arnold WJ, Rothschild EW, et al, Tidal Irrigation Cooperating Group. Tidal irrigation versus conservative medical management in patients with osteoarthritis of the knee: a prospective randomized study. J Rheumatol 1992;19:772–9.

[5] Livesley PJ, Doherty M, Needoff M, et al. Arthroscopic lavage of osteoarthritic knees. J Bone Joint Surg Br 1991;73:922–6.

[6] Gibson JN, White MD, Chapman VM, et al. Arthroscopic lavage and debridement for osteoarthritis of the knee. J Bone Joint Surg Br 1992;74(4):534–7.

[7] Magnuson PB. Joint debridement, surgical treatment of degenerative arthritis. Surg Gynecol Obstet 1941;73:1–9.

[8] Pridie KH. Method of resurfacing osteoarthritic knee joints. J Bone Joint Surg Br 1959;41:618–9.

[9] Jackson RW, Dieterichs C. The results of arthroscopic lavage and debridement of osteoarthritic knees based on the severity of degeneration: a 4- to 6-year symptomatic follow-up. Arthroscopy 2003;19(1):13–20.

[10] Outerbridge RE. The etiology of chondromalacia patellae. 1961. Clin Orthop Relat Res 2001;389:5–8.

[11] Chambers K, Schulzer M, Sobolev B, et al. Degenerative arthritis arthroscopy and research. J Arthroscopy 2002;18:686–7.

[12] Hubbard MJ. Articular debridement versus washout for degeneration of the medial femoral condyle. A five-year study. J Bone Joint Surg Br 1996;78:217–9.

[13] Merchan EC, Galindo E. Arthroscope-guided surgery versus nonoperative treatment for limited degenerative osteoarthritis of the femorotibial joint in patients over 50 years of age: a prospective comparative study. Arthroscopy 1993;9(6):663–7.

[14] Fond J, Rudin D, Ahmad S, et al. Arthroscopic debridement of osteoarthritis of the knee: 2- and 5-year results. Arthroscopy 2002;18:829–34.

[15] Bonamo JJ, Kessler KJ, et al. Arthroscopic meniscectomy in patients over the age of 40. Am J Sports Med 1992;20(4):422–8 [discussion 428–9].

[16] Pearse EO, Craig DM. Partial meniscectomy in the presence of severe osteoarthritis does not hasten the symptomatic progression of osteoarthritis. Arthroscopy 2003;19:963–8.

[17] Jones RE, Smith EC, Reisch JS. Effects of medial meniscectomy in patients older than 40 years. J Bone Joint Surg Am 1978;60:783–6.

[18] Puddu G, Cipolla M, Cerullo G, et al. Arthroscopic treatment of the flexed arthritic knee in active middle-aged patients. Knee Surg Sports Traumatol Arthrosc 1994;2:73–5.

[19] Aichroth PM, Patel DV, Moyes ST. A prospective review of arthroscopic debridement for degenerative joint disease of the knee. Int Orthop 1991;15:351–5.

[20] Boldin C, Fankhauser F, Seibert FJ, et al. Arthroscopy of total knee arthroplasties: indications and technical problems. European Surgery 2002;34(5):309–11.

[21] Bert JM, Maschka K. The arthroscopic treatment of unicompartmental gonarthrosis: a five-year follow-up study of abrasion arthroplasty plus arthroscopic debridement and arthroscopic debridement alone. Arthroscopy 1989;5(1):25–32.

[22] Sprague III NF. Arthroscopic debridement for degenerative knee joint disease. Clin Orthop Relat Res 1981;160:118–23.

[23] Rand JA. Arthroscopic management of degenerative meniscus tears in patients with degenerative arthritis. Arthroscopy 1985;1:253–8.

[24] Ogilvie-Harris DJ, Fitsialos BP. Arthroscopic management of the degenerative knee. Arthroscopy 1991;7:151–7.

[25] Segal L, Day SE, Chapman AB, et al. Can we reduce disease burden from osteoarthritis? Med J Aust 2004;180(Suppl 5):S11–7.

ELSEVIER
SAUNDERS

Orthop Clin N Am 36 (2005) 419–426

A Treatment Algorithm for the Management of Articular Cartilage Defects

Jason M. Scopp, MD[a],*, Bert R. Mandelbaum, MD[b]

[a]Peninsula Orthopaedic Associates, 111 Davis Street, Salisbury, MD 21804, USA
[b]Santa Monica Orthopaedic and Sports Medicine Group, 1301 20th Street, Suite 150, Santa Monica, CA 90404, USA

In 1743, Hunter [1] described ulcerations of articular cartilage as problems that will not heal. The clinical consequences of articular cartilage defects of the knee are pain, swelling, mechanical symptoms, athletic and functional disability, and osteoarthritis (OA) (Fig. 1). Full thickness articular cartilage defects have a poor capacity to heal. The challenge to restore the articular cartilage surface is multidimensional, faced by basic scientists in the laboratory and orthopedic surgeons in the operating room. This article provides an overview of the contemporary treatment options available for the restoration of articular cartilage defects of the knee.

The evolution of cartilage repair options

Full thickness articular cartilage injury incites a limited intrinsic healing response. This response begins with hematoma formation, stem cell migration, and vascular ingrowth [2]. The response usually produces type I collagen resulting in fibrocartilage rather than the preferred hyaline cartilage that is produced by the chondrocyte [3]. This "repair cartilage" has diminished resilience and stiffness with poor wear characteristics. The first attempted

articular cartilage repair techniques employed procedures that included lavage and debridement, and drilling or microfracture to stimulate mesenchymal stem cell metaplasia to form fibrocartilage. Newer substitution replacement techniques use either autograft or allograft to fill defects in articular cartilage. Most recent technologies involve biologic replacement techniques using autologous chondrocyte cell culture technology (Fig. 2).

Mesenchymal stem cell stimulation: abrasion arthroplasty and microfracture

Abrasion arthroplasty is performed using a shaver or a burr to remove the superficial 1 to 2 mm of sclerotic subchondral bone to expose the underlying vascular subchondral plate [4]. The violation of the subchondral vasculature allows a clot to form within the defect that later develops into fibrocartilage. Jackson and colleagues [5] in 1988 and Jackson [6] in 1991 demonstrated initial improvement with this technique, but these results deteriorate over time.

Microfracture involves penetrating the subchondral bone to expose the articular cartilage defect to pluripotent marrow stem cells (Fig. 3). The mesenchymal stem cell derived from bone marrow can differentiate along a chondrogenic lineage [7,8]. Microfracture is favored over abrasion arthroplasty because it is less destructive to the subchondral bone and has a higher degree of controlled depth penetration. Microfracture has been shown to increase

* Corresponding author.
E-mail address: JscoppMD@PeninsulaOrtho.com
(J.M. Scopp).

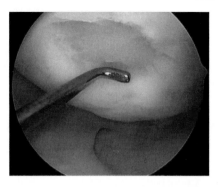

Fig. 1. Arthroscopic picture depicting a full-thickness, grade IV articular cartilage defect of the medial femoral condyle.

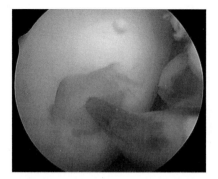

Fig. 3. Arthroscopic picture of the microfracture technique of a medial femoral condyle articular cartilage defect.

the tissue volume and percentage of type 2 collagen in filling defects when compared with untreated defects [9].

Substitution replacement options

Lexer [10] first introduced the repair of osteo-chondral defects by segmental replacement with fresh allografts in 1908. In a study of segmental allograft replacement for large traumatic articular cartilage defects, McDermott and colleagues [11] reported good or excellent results in 75% and 64% of their patients at 5 and 10 years, respectively. Ghazavi and colleagues [12] demonstrated 95% survival at 5 years, 71% at 10 years, and 66% at 20 years. Although these results have stood the test of time, the logistical problems of tissue procurement by using fresh, un-irradiated osteochondral grafts coupled with the potential for disease transmission have limited the widespread application of these techniques.

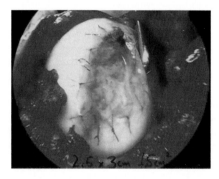

Fig. 2. This is a medial femoral condyle lesion that has undergone microsuturing of a periosteal patch with implantation of cultured autologous chondrocytes.

Autograft substitution replacements have become popular for the management of articular cartilage defects. Initially studied in a dog model, Hangody [13] reported on osteochondral plug repair of articular cartilage defects. He demonstrated survival of the osteohyaline plug while the interstices filled with fi-brocartilage. The advantage of autograft replacement solves the logistical problems inherent in the use of allografts. However, autograft replacement cannot be used for large defects and is associated with donor site morbidity. Autograft replacement may also result in abnormal stress–strain distributions in articular cartilage [14].

Cell/biologic replacement options

In 1989, Grande and colleagues [15] demonstrated in a rabbit model a more complete repair of articular defects when periosteal transplants were supplemented with cultured chondrocytes. The rationale for this procedure is based on the ability of normal articular chondrocytes to dedifferentiate in monolayer culture and undergo proliferative expansion [16]. This expansion provides a large number of cells that can be transferred into a large articular cartilage defect; the cells are contained by a periosteal flap where they differentiate and make hyaline-like cartilage (Fig. 4).

In 2002, Peterson and colleagues [17] evaluated the biomechanics and long-term durability of autologous chondrocyte implantation. Using an electro-mechanical indentation probe during second-look arthroscopies, the investigators demonstrated stiffness measurements of 90% or more when compared with adjacent normal articular cartilage. Briggs and colleagues [18] demonstrated histologically the potential to express type IIa and type IIb collagen in 14 of

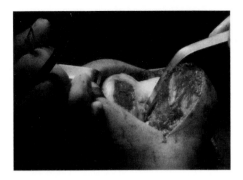

Fig. 4. Intraoperative photograph of periosteal patch placement before microsuturing during autologous chondrocyte implantation.

14 patients, and saw regenerated hyaline cartilage in 8 of 14 patients.

Reoperation after autologous chondrocyte implantation is indicated when mechanical symptoms develop. The most common reason for the development of these symptoms is periosteal hypertrophy [19]. Henderson and colleagues [19] reoperated on 22 of 135 patients treated with autologous chondrocyte implantation for knee pain or mechanical symptoms at a mean 10.5 months after surgery. Of the 31 grafted lesions, 30 had normal or near-normal visual repair scores, and biopsy showed good integration with subchondral bone and at the marginal interface.

Clinical management

The clinical management of articular cartilage defects depends on several factors. Although the progression of a symptomatic lesion has been well demonstrated, the natural history of an asymptomatic lesion is unknown [20]. As a consequence, the clinician must define, characterize, and classify local, regional, and systemic, medical, and family history factors that may influence the progression, degeneration, or regeneration of the defect.

Local and regional factors

To ensure uniform standards of evaluating articular cartilage repair, a universally accepted classification system is necessary. The International Cartilage Repair Society (ICRS) has developed a comprehensive method of documentation and classi-

fication [21]. The following variables are included in the standards:

- Etiology: Is the defect acute or chronic? This differentiation may be difficult because many injuries are acute on chronic.
- Defect thickness: What is the thickness or depth of the defect as defined by the ICRS grade? (Fig. 3). Penetration of the tidemark or the presence of subchondral cysts can affect the functional articular cartilage unit.
- Lesion size: A probe accurately measures size in centimeters squared during arthroscopy. Defects less than 2 cm^2 have different treatment options from defects greater than 2 cm^2.
- Degree of containment: Is the defect contained or uncontained? Is the surrounding articular cartilage healthy or degenerative? As the degree of containment decreases, consequent loss of joint space is seen on radiographs (Fig. 5).
- Location: Is the defect in the weight-bearing region of the knee? Is it monopolar or bipolar?
- Ligamentous integrity: Are the cruciate ligaments intact, partially torn, or completely torn? Is there residual instability or has the knee been reconstructed?
- Meniscal integrity: Are the menisci intact? If not, has there been a partial, subtotal, or complete meniscectomy? Has meniscal repair or transplantation been performed?
- Alignment: Is the alignment normal, varus, or valgus? Is there patellofemoral malalignment? Has an osteotomy or realignment procedure been performed?
- Previous management: If a prior cartilage restorative procedure has been performed, was the subchondral plate violated?
- Radiologic assessment: Weight-bearing anteroposterior (AP) or flexed posteroanterior (PA), lateral, and patellofemoral views are necessary for the evaluation of joint-space narrowing and subchondral cyst formation.
- MRI assessment: New MRI sequences allow for the preoperative and postoperative evaluation of defects and articular cartilage repairs. Bone bruising, osteochondritis dissecans, and avascular necrosis can also be evaluated (Fig. 6).
- General medical, systemic, and family history issues: Is there a rheumatologic history? Are there endocrine related factors? Is there a family history of OA or cartilage disorders?

A comprehensive analysis of the local and regional factors related to an articular cartilage lesion is

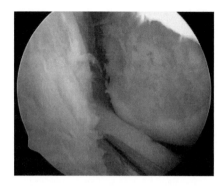

Fig. 5. A large uncontained grade IV defect of the lateral trochlea in a patient who has patellofemoral instability.

used to develop a treatment plan. A flow chart has been created to summarize primary treatment options and secondary treatment options. There are separate charts for femoral and for patellar defects. Primary treatment options should be considered first-line treatment choices. Secondary treatment options are considered if primary treatment fails or if other factors prevent the use of a primary treatment option (Figs. 7 and 8).

It is imperative to consider each lesion in the context of alignment, ligamentous, and meniscal integrity (macroenvironment). Similarly, the micro-environment must also be considered. The micro-environment of the knee is a term used to describe the molecular level factors (chondrocyte function, synovium, chondropenia) that influence cartilage integrity.

The clinical algorithm: the chondropenic pathway

After completion of the comprehensive assessment, patients can then be stratified in a clinical algorithm. This chondropenic pathway has been developed for the management of articular cartilage defects. The algorithm defines ten patient-directed situations based on lesion size, depth, and associated issues such as alignment, ligament, and meniscal integrity. Each situation considers the problem category, the therapeutic options, and the current unresolved issues.

Situation No. 1

Problem

Meniscus tears and partial-thickness articular cartilage defects. (This is the most common condition the orthopedic surgeon sees in practice.)

Therapeutic options

Arthroscopic debridement and partial meniscectomy followed by rehabilitation physical and conditioning therapy.

Unresolved issues

Role of radiofrequency probes. Do they cause chondrocyte death or decrease regenerative and more degenerative or avascular consequences (bipolar, monopolar)? Why and when to use glucosamine and chondroitin sulfate and viscosupplementation?

Situation No. 2

Problem

Femoral articular cartilage defects less than 1 cm^2.

Therapeutic options

Debridement, microfracture, osteochondral grafting.

Unresolved issues

Do small defects heal sufficiently well in the short- and long-term with mesenchymal stem-cell stimulation techniques such as microfracture?

Situation No. 3

Problem

Femoral articular cartilage defects, including osteochondritis dissecans size 1 to 2 cm^2.

Therapeutic primary options

Debridement, microfracture, osteochondral grafting, and autologous chondrocyte implantation.

Therapeutic secondary options

Osteochondral grafting and autologous chondrocyte implantation.

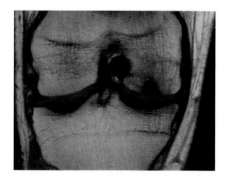

Fig. 6. A nonenhanced magnetic resonance image of an articular cartilage defect of the medial femoral condyle.

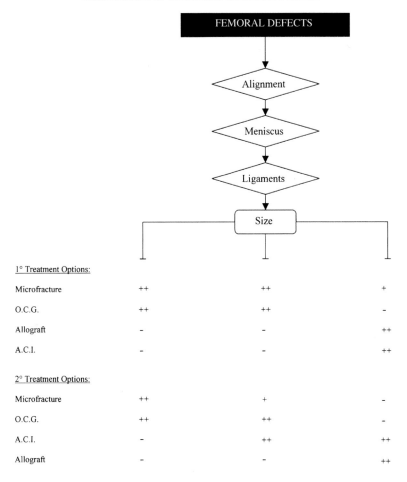

Fig. 7. Flowchart demonstrating the primary and secondary treatment algorithm for isolated femoral condyle defects. For each defect, appropriate treatment is staged to avoid compromise of postoperative rehabilitation. Treatment was either not recommended (−), acceptable (+), or optimal (++). ACI, autologous chondrocyte implantation; OCG, osteochondral graft.

Unresolved issues
Is a mesenchymal stem-cell stimulation technique an acceptable primary option?

Situation No. 4

Problem
Femoral articular cartilage defects, including osteochondritis dissecans greater than 2 cm^2 (Fig. 9).

Therapeutic primary options
Autologous chondrocyte implantation and fresh allograft.

Therapeutic secondary options
Autologous chondrocyte implantation and fresh allograft.

Unresolved issues
What is the optimal and maximal size of lesion to which osteochondral autografts can be applied?

Situation No. 5

Problem
Complex femoral articular defects with malalignment, ligament, or meniscal deficiency.

Therapeutic primary options
Osteotomy, meniscal repair or allograft, cruciate reconstructions, autologous chondrocyte implantation, fresh allograft, or osteochondral autograft depending on size.

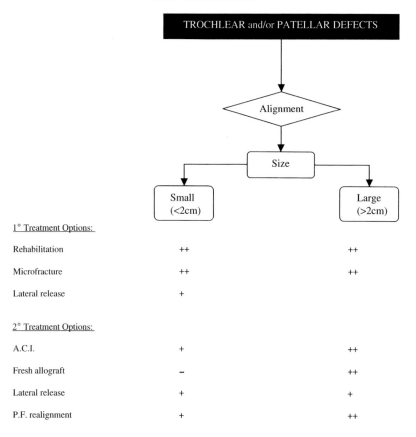

	Small (<2cm)	Large (>2cm)
1° Treatment Options:		
Rehabilitation	++	++
Microfracture	++	++
Lateral release	+	
2° Treatment Options:		
A.C.I.	+	++
Fresh allograft	–	++
Lateral release	+	+
P.F. realignment	+	++

Fig. 8. Flowchart demonstrating the primary and secondary treatment algorithm for patellar and trochlear defects. Treatment was either not recommended (−), acceptable (+), or optimal (++).

Unresolved issues

How to optimally stage procedures so that index postoperative protocol does not compromise integrity of secondary or tertiary procedures. Which meniscus allograft, osteotomies, or ligament reconstruction procedure to use?

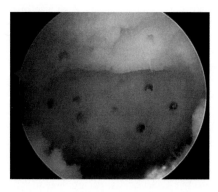

Fig. 9. A large osteochondral defect of the medial femoral condyle surrounded by grade IV articular cartilage changes. (Note: drilling and microfracture have been performed.)

Situation No. 6

Problem

Patellar or trochlear articular cartilage defects with no malalignment or instability.

Therapeutic primary options

Physical and conditioning therapy, including tapping bracing and pelvic stabilization.

Therapeutic secondary options

Arthroscopy and lateral release, therapeutic tertiary options, autologous chondrocyte implantation plus anteromedialization or patellofemoral realignment osteotomy.

Unresolved issues

What are the definitive indications for arthroscopic lateral release? Does viscosupplementation have a role early in management of patellofemoral chondromalacia syndrome?

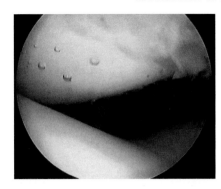

Fig. 10. Arthroscopic image of patellofemoral malalignment manifest by patellar contacting the lateral trochlea.

Situation No. 7

Problem

Patellar and trochlear articular cartilage defects, with significant malalignment or instability (Fig. 10).

Therapeutic primary options

Physical and conditioning therapy, including tapping bracing and pelvic stabilization.

Therapeutic secondary options

Autologous chondrocyte implantation plus anteromedialization or patellofemoral realignment osteotomy.

Unresolved issues

Is the role of osteotomy beneficial early on to disease modifying such that it will prevent OA of the patellofemoral joint?

Situation No. 8

Problem

Tibial articular cartilage defects, with no significant malalignment or instability.

Therapeutic options

Osteotomy as required in relation to the degree of malalignment in combination with microfracture or autologous chondrocyte implantation depending on size of lesion.

Unresolved issues

Successful access may require release of collateral ligaments and detached meniscus insertions. Concomitant procedures protocols should not conflict with postoperative rehabilitative protocol.

Situation No. 9

Problem

Significant chondropenia and early OA (global grade III/IV articular cartilage defects in the 30- to 60-year-old patient who has degenerative meniscal tears) (Fig. 11).

Therapeutic options

Nonsteroidal anti-inflammatory medications/Cox-2 inhibitors; hyaluronic acid; glucosamine/chondroitin sulfate; bike for exercise; unloading braces; arthroscopy for mechanical symptoms, loose bodies, and meniscal tears; and osteotomy selectively as required in relation to the degree of malalignment or joint-space narrowing.

Unresolved issues

Is there a role for biologic resurfacing procedures concomitant with realignment procedures?

Situation No. 10

Problem

Degenerative meniscal tears and global grade IV defects (late OA).

Therapeutic options

Nonsteroidal anti-inflammatory medications/ Cox-2 inhibitors; hyaluronic acid; glucosamine/ chondroitin sulfate; bike for exercise; unloading braces; arthroscopy for mechanical symptoms, loose bodies, and meniscal tears; osteotomy selectively as required in relation to the degree of malalignment or joint-space narrowing; and total knee arthroplasty.

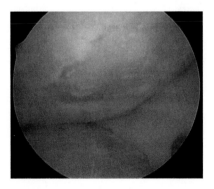

Fig. 11. Bipolar grade IV lesions (femoral and tibial) with meniscus pathology.

Unresolved issues

What is the role of arthroscopy in late OA other than alleviation of mechanical symptoms?

Summary and future challenges

The challenges of articular cartilage repair and restoration continue despite recent advances. Marrow stimulation techniques, substitution replacement options, and biologic replacement options each have a role in the treatment algorithm of articular cartilage defects. Yet no single treatment option can reestablish the hyaline cartilage seen in normal articular cartilage. The goal, then, is to develop new technologies and disease-modifying interventions that protect and preserve the joint over time by maintaining biochemical, biomechanical, and cellular integrity. Until these technologies exist, collaboration between the basic scientist and the clinician will continue to advance the current technologies in an effort to restore the violated articular cartilage surface.

References

[1] Hunter W. Of the structure and diseases of articulating cartilages. Philos Trans R Soc Lond B Biol Sci 1743; 42B:514–21.

[2] Buckwalter JA, Rosenberg LC, Hunziker EB. Articular cartilage: composition, structure, response to injury and methods of facilitating repair. In: Ewing JW, editor. Articular cartilage and knee joint function: basic science and arthroscopy. New York: Raven Press; 1990. p. 19–56.

[3] Furukawa T, Eyre DR, Koide S, et al. Biomechanical studies on repair cartilage resurfacing experimental defects in the rabbit knee. J Bone Joint Surg Am 1980; 62:79–89.

[4] Johnson LL. Arthroscopic abrasion arthroplasty. Historical and pathologic perspective: present status. Arthroscopy 1986;2:54–69.

[5] Jackson RW, Marans HJ, Silver RS. Arthroscopic treatment of degenerative arthritis of the knee. J Bone Joint Surg Br 1988;70:332–6.

[6] Jackson RW. Arthroscopic treatment of degenerative arthritis. In: McGinty JB, editor. Operative arthroscopy. New York: Raven Press; 1991. p. 319–23.

[7] Barry FP. Mesenchymal stem cell differentiation in vitro along chondrogenic lines. Trans Orthop Res Soc 1997;22:222–8.

[8] Johnstone LL, Yoo JU, Barry FP. In vitro chondrogenesis of marrow-derived mesenchymal cells. Trans Orthop Res Soc 1997;21:65.

[9] Frisbee DD, Trotter GW, Powers BE, et al. Arthroscopic subchondral bone plate microfracture technique augments healing of large chondral defects in the radial carpal bone and medial femoral condyle of horses. Vet Surg 1999;28:242–55.

[10] Lexer E. Substitution of whole or half joints from freshly amputated extremities by free plastic operation. Surg Gynecol Obstet 1908;6:601–7.

[11] McDermott AGP, Langer F, Pritzker KPH, et al. Fresh small-fragment osteochondral allografts: long-term follow-up study on first 100 cases. Clin Orthop 1985; 197:96–102.

[12] Ghazavi MT, Pritzker KP, Davis AM, et al. Fresh osteochondral allografts for post-traumatic osteochondritis dissecans of the knee. J Bone Joint Surg Br 1997; 79:1008–13.

[13] Hangody L, Kish G, Kárpáti Z, et al. Autogenous osteochondral graft technique for replacing knee cartilage defects in dogs. Orthopedics Int 1997;5:175–81.

[14] Wu JZ, Herzog W, Hasler EM. Inadequate placement of osteochondral plugs may induce abnormal stressstrain distributions in articular cartilage—finite element simulations. Med Eng Phys 2002;24(2):85–97.

[15] Grande DA, Pitman MI, Peterson L, et al. The repair of experimentally produced defects in rabbit articular cartilage by autologous chondrocyte implantation. J Orthop Res 1989;7:208–18.

[16] Benya PD, Schaffer JD. Dedifferentiated chondrocytes reexpress the differentiated collagen phenotype when cultured in agarose gels. Cell 1982;30:215–24.

[17] Peterson L, Brittberg M, Kiviranta I, et al. Autologous chondrocyte transplantation. Biomechanics and longterm durability. Am J Sports Med 2002;30:2–12.

[18] Briggs TW, Mahroof S, David LA, et al. Histological evaluation of chondral defects after autologous chondrocyte implantation of the knee. J Bone Joint Surg Br 2003;85(7):1077–83.

[19] Henderson I, Tuy B, Oakes B. Reoperation after autologous chondrocyte implantation. Indications and findings. J Bone Joint Surg Br 2004;86(2):205–11.

[20] Shelbourne KD, Jari S, Gray T. Outcome of untreated traumatic traumatic articlular cartilage defects of the knee: a natural history study. J Bone Joint Surg Am 2003;85(Suppl 2):8–16.

[21] International Cartilage Repair Society Cartilage Injury Evaluation Package. Developed during ICRS 2000 Standards Workshop. Schloss Munchenwiler, Switzerland, January 27–30, 2000.

ELSEVIER
SAUNDERS

Orthop Clin N Am 36 (2005) 427–431

ORTHOPEDIC
CLINICS
OF NORTH AMERICA

Radiofrequency Use on Articular Cartilage Lesions

C. Thomas Vangsness, Jr, MD

Department of Orthopaedic Surgery, Keck School of Medicine, University of Southern California, 1520 San Pablo Street, Suite 2000, Los Angeles, CA 90033, USA

The incidence of knee arthritis is increasing in our society and presents many dilemmas to the patient and doctor. Recent advances in arthroscopic treatment of arthritis have lead to the development of radiofrequency energy as an adjunctive tool for many arthroscopic procedures [1,2]. Of great concern is the recent use of radiofrequency energy to treat articular cartilage lesions in the knee.

Published reports have documented the problems associated with the use of thermal energy on articular cartilage, especially lasers [3–5]. Reviewing publications concerning in vitro and in vivo evaluations of the use of radiofrequency devices on articular cartilage creates confusion for the orthopedic surgeon. Close scrutiny of study design creates a strong concern for the indiscriminate use of radiofrequency energy in treating articular cartilage lesions in the knee. The testing parameters needed to evaluate radiofrequency energy are diverse and need to be specifically controlled. The popularity of thermal chondroplasty is a challenge to the orthopedic surgeon.

Basic science studies

Kaplan and colleagues [6] investigated the acute effects of bipolar radiofrequency energy on fresh human articular cartilage. The depth of radiofrequency penetration increased with increasing power settings. Using six fresh human explants, they concluded that "radiofrequency was safe for use on articular cartilage." Unfortunately, this study did not

strictly control the degenerative status of the tested human articular cartilage and the parameters under which the energy was delivered. The histology tests were conducted with hemotoxin and eosin (H&E) staining techniques, which are not as accurate as confocal laser microscopy [7,8]. Therefore, firm conclusions cannot be made from this in vitro study.

Turner and colleagues [9] examined radiofrequency use versus a mechanical shaver with an in vivo model using sheep. They found bipolar radiofrequency to be superior histologically to mechanical debridement of knee cartilage at 24 weeks. Unfortunately, the hand application of the radiofrequency energy was not specifically controlled, and extrapolation of this data to human use should not be made.

Edwards and colleagues [10] compared bipolar versus monopolar radiofrequency devices in an in vitro "chondromalacic" human cartilage study. They found greater penetration with bipolar than monopolar energy using controlled microscopy. Again, strict application of radiofrequency energy was not controlled with manual radiofrequency energy application in this study. Lu and colleagues [7] evaluated bipolar energy on human articular cartilage and compared confocal laser microscopy with light microscopy. They found bipolar radiofrequency penetrated deeper into human articular cartilage than monopolar radiofrequency. Again, this study did not use strict control of this delivery of energy.

More recent work by Lu and colleagues [11] and Amiel and colleagues [12] have investigated radiofrequency generator, power control, and probe design to limit the chondrocyte death. The study by Lu and colleagues using a ceramic insulated probe caused less chondrocyte damage than the tested monopolar or bipolar radiofrequency probes. The study by Amiel

E-mail address: vangsnes@usc.edu

doi:10.1016/j.ocl.2005.05.002

orthopedic.theclinics.com

and colleagues showed that the radiofrequency energy cell death had no significant effects on the metabolic activity of the remaining cartilage.

Studies have evaluated the temperature and effect of the arthroscopic lavage solution. Temperature and treatment duration can affect the delivered temperature of the radiofrequency energy to the tissue (increased solution temperature gave less energy transfer). The arthroscopic solution flow rate appeared to have less of an effect on energy transfer and tissue damage [13–16].

Another study by Lu and colleagues [17] reported on negative effects of monopolar radiofrequency energy and partial defects in using the sheep model. The authors concluded that monopolar radiofrequency energy caused immediate chondrocyte death and influenced proteoglycan concentration. They caution against using radiofrequency imaging for chondroplasty.

Yet another study by Lu and colleagues [18] investigated bipolar and monopolar devices with an in vitro bovine articular cartilage study. They applied a motorized jig with 50 g of weight to the probe tip at a velocity of 1 mm/s. They compared this with a manual "paintbrush" clinical application. They looked at three different commercial devices and found that the bipolar radiofrequency energy device contoured the articular cartilage significantly faster than the monopolar. Chondrocyte death was greater with the bipolar radiofrequency energy systems when compared with the monopolar in all tested specimens. The investigators concluded that in using the manufacturers' recommended settings, immediate chondrocyte death was noticed especially in the bipolar systems. In many cases the death extended down to the subchondral bone. The investigators cautioned about the use of radiofrequency energy with thermal chondroplasty.

Edwards and colleagues [10] took chondromalacic cartilage (grade II & III) from patients undergoing total knee arthroplasty. Using three standard radiofrequency commercial products at manufacturers' recommended settings with a custom designed jig and controlling the irrigation flow of saline at 22°C, they found that all three radiofrequency devices successfully smoothed the chondromalacic cartilage surfaces. Bipolar devices gave significantly greater chondrocyte death than monopolar. Chondrocyte death went to the level of the subchondral bone in over 50% of the tested samples with the bipolar devices when compared with the monopolar devices. The investigators felt that monopolar and bipolar radiofrequency devices were potentially unsafe for human chondroplasty.

Edwards and colleagues [13] evaluated bipolar and monopolar radiofrequency energy in a study examining cartilage matrix temperatures at three depths below the articular surface. Fresh bovine osteochondral sections had a guided floral optic thermal couple placed at 200, 500, and 2000 μm below the articular surface. They found that cartilage temperatures were significantly higher in the bipolar radiofrequency group than the monopolar radiofrequency group at all depths. Bipolar energy temperatures were consistently greater than those of monopolar energy at the three measured depths of articular cartilage. At 200 μm and 500 μm below the articular cartilage surface, temperatures of bipolar radiofrequency energy exceeded 75°C, whereas the monopolar radiofrequency energy exceeded 50°. Thermal energy is deleterious to the viability of chondrocytes. Chondrocyte death can occur at 45°C to 55°C [19–21].

Lu and colleagues [22] investigated radiofrequency energy treatment time with chondrocyte viability and surface contouring using fresh grade II human articular cartilage lesions. Using monopolar and bipolar radiofrequency devices with a custom designed jig at six different intervals, they found that frons of articular cartilage were "melted" with radiofrequency energy and macroscopic smoothing was noted. The six intervals ranged from 5 seconds to 40 seconds and scanning electron microscopy demonstrated that monopolar radiofrequency energy and bipolar radiofrequency energy contoured rough chondromalacic surfaces, depending on the treatment times. The study showed that bipolar radiofrequency energy caused significantly greater chondrocyte death than monopolar energy for each treatment interval. Again, the investigators noted that thermal chondroplasty can cause significant chondrocyte death. Unfortunately, this study did not control the application force of these radiofrequency devices on the articular cartilage surfaces, which biased their result.

Ryan and colleagues [23] tested equine cartilage with bipolar radiofrequency at three different power settings. Proteoglycan and chondrocyte degradation increased with increased power settings on fibrillated cartilage with hand application of radiofrequency energy.

Cook and colleagues [24] looked at monopolar and bipolar radiofrequency energy applied to human knee cartilage explants and documented a change in stiffness and H & E staining with different radiofrequency energy levels. They documented significant cell death and macroscopic smoothing of the articular cartilage surface.

Lu and colleagues [11] presented work using an in vitro bovine cartilage model to evaluate monopolar and bipolar probes with an emphasis on a newer monopolar ceramic insulated probe tip. Confocal microscopy demonstrated that the ceramic probe produced less chondrocyte death compared with the standard monopolar and bipolar probes tested.

Edwards and colleagues [25] recently presented an in vivo equine study comparing a ceramic monopolar radiofrequency probe with mechanical debridement and a commercially available bipolar radiofrequency energy for patellar chondroplasty procedures. The 6-months follow-up showed the new monopolar ceramic probe contoured the cartilage surface better than mechanical debridement and maintained thicker cartilage compared with the mechanical debridement and the bipolar radiofrequency device. Also noted was the stiffness in the prototype monopolar radiofrequency device compared with the mechanical device, the bipolar device, and controls.

Caffey and colleagues [26] set up a study with fresh human articular cartilage samples to rigidly control all variables and analyzed the effects of the five commercially available radiofrequency probes in a strictly controlled laboratory setting. Simulating operating room conditions, the investigators attached five commercially available radiofrequency probes to a customized jig to standardize the contact pressure for each investigated probe at the articular cartilage surface. The cartilage samples were kept refrigerated in a phosphate-buffered saline (PBS) solution and tested the same day. The investigators evaluated grade II articular cartilage and some grade III cartilage lesions from human femoral condyles. A minimal perpendicular contact pressure of 2 g stabilized the probe tip against the articular cartilage surfaces in a 37°C bath. This study was setup to deliver a minimal amount of radiofrequency energy to fresh articular cartilage. The study included five current radiofrequency generators and their manufactures' most current radiofrequency probes at the time of the experiments, without any industrial financial support. The investigators randomly and blindly tested each probe. Radiofrequency energy treatment times were 1 second and 3 seconds for 15 cartilage specimens from ten different patients. All testing and imaging was done immediately after harvesting, and confocal microscopy imaging was done after waiting 3 hours after radiofrequency treatment. The investigators tested and evaluated a total of 109 grade II samples and 15 type III cartilage specimens, and conducted t-tests to compare the mean maximal cell deaths between each radiofrequency device at 1 and 3 seconds of application times. Using confocal microscopy, the maximum average cell death was 479 μm and 1124 μm for treatment times of 1 second and 3 seconds, respectively. All the probes yielded a well-demarcated half-circle border between the chondrocytes (brightly stained with calcein green) and an area just above the border that was devoid of all living chondrocytes (Fig. 1). The one radiofrequency probe that was recommended to be kept 1 mm off the articular cartilage surface did not demonstrate any distinguishable area of cellular death at the manufacturer's setting under these testing parameters. All the grade III cartilage specimens tested showed cell death down to bone. All contacting probes removed fibrillation of the articular cartilage in the treatment area. In setting up the design of the experiments, several attempts to control "light" hand pressure with the probe gave inconsistent changes and a wide variability of cartilage cell death. This inconsistency and variability led to using a specifically designed jig to hold the radiofrequency probe for consistent and reproducible energy application. Using the current recommendations of the five radiofrequency companies, no significant differences between the mean depths of monopolar or bipolar devices at 1-second treatment time or 3-second treatment time were found. Under these rigidly controlled conditions and using fresh human grade II human articular cartilage, no difference was observed between the monopolar and the bipolar probes. As the depth of femoral articular cartilage has been reported to be 1.65 to 2.6 mm [27], approximately 18% to 29% of the articular cartilage thickness at the site of 1 second application and 42% to 68% of the articular cartilage thickness at 3 seconds of radiofrequency application were destroyed under these minimal energy conditions and parameters.

This study demonstrated that manual application of radiofrequency probes was inaccurate when

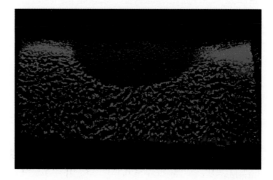

Fig. 1. Confocal microscopy slide of articular cartilage. In this hemisection, red shows the dead cells and green the viable cells after radiofrequency energy application.

attempting to control administration of heat. The generator temperature–sensing feedback regulators used to control radiofrequency probes have been shown to be inaccurate [20,28,29]. Visual feedback for radiofrequency energy application also has been shown to be inaccurate with a delayed "thermal latency" effect observed after the generator has been turned off [20,28,30]. Under these most minimal of thermal conditions, this study reinforced the lack of feedback the surgeon has regarding the temperature and energy delivered to the cartilage during surgery.

Application of radiofrequency heat to grade III cartilage can easily remove all cartilage cells and transmit energy to subchondral bone. The thermal effect on subchondral bone is a major concern and is not well understood [3,31]. This study cautioned against overheating articular cartilage and did not recommend the use of these radiofrequency probes.

Human clinical studies

To date, there are two published human trials investigating radiofrequency energy on articular cartilage. Owens and colleagues [32] prospectively evaluated bipolar radiofrequency energy versus a standard mechanical shaver blade in 39 consecutive patients who had a grade II-III patellar articular cartilage lesion. They applied energy to debride the cartilage by hand using nonablative energy parameters for an uncertain duration of time. At 2 years, using a new patellofemoral joint evaluation scoring system, they found a statistical improvement in patient outcome with the use of bipolar radiofrequency energy on these isolated patellar chondral lesions.

In a randomized double-blind prospective study, Stein and colleagues [33] treated 146 patients who had mechanical chondroplasty or mechanical chondroplasty and electrocautery to "smooth the lesions." The wand was hand-held 1 to 2 mm off the surface of the cartilage at 40 W for an uncertain amount of time. At 12-months follow-up, they found no significant differences in the patients who had grade II lesions, though grade III lesions favored the control, non-radiofrequency treatment group. The investigators felt that electrocautery as an adjunct to chondroplasty offered little benefit to chondromalacic lesions and may limit successful outcomes.

Summary

As many of the published in vitro and in vivo studies using animal and human articular cartilage

demonstrate, the cartilage effects of radiofrequency energy are confounding and difficult to interpret. Most of the studies have not adequately controlled the many variables necessary to establish the science in the area of radiofrequency chondroplasty.

The main purpose for radiofrequency probes is to generate and deliver heat to targeted cells [2,34]. The heat generated within the saline environment during arthroscopy injures the chondrocytes. Because of the excessive fragility of chondrocytes and their known inability to regenerate, it is important to limit any unnecessary heat to articular cartilage cells, as chondrocytes die at temperatures of 45°C to 55°C [19–21].

Current opinions regarding the use of radiofrequency energy for the treatment of articular cartilage lesions are diverse and contradictory. There are many variables that have not been clearly defined when investigating radiofrequency use, and it is essential that these variables are specifically defined to gather appropriate scientific conclusions for clinical use during surgery. The orthopedic surgeon should understand these issues and attempt to preserve articular cartilage cells at all times. The literature lacks evidence-based medicine and randomized clinical trials to make any accurate statement about the clinical use of RF energy on articular cartilage.

References

[1] Edwards RB, Markel M. Radiofrequency energy treatment effects on articular cartilage. Operative Techniques in Orthopaedics 2001;11:96–104.
[2] Polousky JD, Hedman TP, Vangsness Jr CT. Electrosurgical methods for arthroscopic meniscectomy: a review of the literature. Arthroscopy 2000;16(8):813–21.
[3] Thal R, Danziger MB, Kelly A. Delayed articular cartilage slough: two cases resulting from holmium: YAG laser damage to normal articular cartilage and a review of the literature. Arthroscopy 1996;12:92–4.
[4] Vangsness Jr CT, Ghaderi B. A literature review of lasers and articular cartilage. Orthopedics 1993;16(5): 593–8.
[5] Vangsness CT, Smith CF, Marshall GJ, et al. CO2 laser vaporization of articular cartilage. Semin Orthop 1992; 7:83–5.
[6] Kaplan L, Uribe JW, Sasken H, et al. The acute effects of radiofrequency energy in articular cartilage: an in vitro study. Arthroscopy 2000;16:2–5.
[7] Lu Y, Edwards III RB, Kalscheur VL, et al. Effect of bipolar radiofrequency energy on human articular cartilage. Comparison of confocal laser microscopy and light microscopy. Arthroscopy 2001;17(2):117–23.
[8] Yetkinler DN, Greenleaf JE, Sherman OH. Histologic analysis of radiofrequency energy chondroplasty. Clin Sports Med 2002;21(4):649–61.

[9] Turner AS, Tippet JW, Powers BE, et al. Radiofrequency (electrosurgical) ablation of articular cartilage: a study in sheep. Arthroscopy 1998;14(6):585–91.

[10] Edwards III RB, Lu Y, Nho S, et al. Thermal chondroplasty of chondromalacic human cartilage. An ex vivo comparison of bipolar and monopolar radiofrequency devices. Am J Sports Med 2002;30:90–7.

[11] Lu Y, Au E, Meyer ML, et al. Prototype radiofrequency probe reduces chondrocyte death compare to current monopolar and bipolar devices for treatment of chondromalacia. Proceedings of the 49th Annual Meeting of Orthopedic Research Society. Elsevier; 2003. p. 688.

[12] Amiel D, Ball ST, Tasto JP. Chondrocyte viability and metabolic activity after treatment of bovine articular cartilage with bipolar radiofrequency: an in vitro study. Arthroscopy 2004;20:503–10.

[13] Edwards III RB, Lu Y, Rodriguez E, et al. Thermometric determination of cartilage matrix temperatures during thermal chondroplasty: comparison of bipolar and monopolar radiofrequency devices. Arthroscopy 2002;18:339–46.

[14] Lu Y, Edwards II RB, Nho S, et al. Lavage solution temperature influences depth of chondrocyte death and surface contouring during thermal chondroplasty with temperature-controlled monopolar radiofrequency energy. Am J Sports Med 2002;30:667–73.

[15] Shellock FG. Radiofrequency energy induced heating of bovine articular cartilage: comparison between temperature-controlled, monopolar, and bipolar systems. Knee Surg Sports Traumatol Arthrosc 2001;9: 392–7.

[16] Shellock FG. Radiofrequency energy-induced heating of bovine cartilage: evaluation of a new temperature-controlled, bipolar radiofrequency system used at different settings. J Knee Surg 2002;15:90–6.

[17] Lu Y, Hayashi K, Hecht P, et al. The effect of monopolar radiofrequency energy on partial-thickness defects of articular cartilage. Arthroscopy 2000;16:527–36.

[18] Lu Y, Edwards III RB, Cole BJ, et al. Thermal chondroplasty with radiofrequency energy. An in vitro comparison of bipolar and monopolar radiofrequency devices. Am J Sports Med 2001;29:42–9.

[19] Kaplan LD, Chu CR, Bradley JP, et al. Recovery of chondrocyte metabolic activity after thermal exposure. Am J Sports Med 2003;31(3):392–8.

[20] Liao WL, Hedman TP, Vangsness Jr CT. Thermal profile of radiofrequency energy in the inferior glenohumeral ligament. Arthroscopy 2004;20(6):603–8.

[21] Wong KL, Williams GR. Complications of thermal capsulorrhaphy of the shoulder. J Bone Joint Surg Am 2001;83:151–5.

[22] Lu Y, Edwards III RB, Nho S, et al. Thermal chondroplasty with bipolar and monopolar radiofrequency energy: effect of treatment time on chondrocyte death and surface contouring. Arthroscopy 2002; 18:779–88.

[23] Ryan A, Bertone A, Kaeding CC, et al. The effects of radiofrequency energy treatment on chondrocytes and matrix of fibrillated articular cartilage. Am J Sports Med 2003;31(3):386–91.

[24] Cook JL, Kuroki K, Kenter K, et al. Bipolar and monopolar radiofrequency treatment of osteoarthritic knee articular cartilage: acute and temporal effects on cartilage compressive stiffness, permeability, cell synthesis, and extracellular matrix composition. J Knee Surg 2004;17(2):99–108.

[25] Edwards RB, Lu Y, Bogdanske JJ, et al. Prototype radiofrequency energy probe stabilizes cartilage matrix in a 6 month in vivo equine model of partial thickness cartilage injury. Proceedings of the 50th Annual Meeting of Orthopedic Research Society. Elsevier; 2004. p. 201.

[26] Caffey S, McPherson E, Moore B, et al. Effects of radiofrequency energy on human articular cartilage: an analysis of five systems. Am J Sports Med 2005;33: 1033–9.

[27] Shepherd DE, Seedhom BB. Thickness of human articular cartilage in joints of the lower limb. Ann Rheum Dis 1999;58:27–34.

[28] Shellock FG, Shields Jr CL. Temperature changes associated with radiofrequency energy-induced heating of bovine capsular tissue: evaluation of bipolar RF electrodes. Arthroscopy 2000;16(4):348–58.

[29] Wickersheim KA, Sun MH. Fluoroptic thermometry. Med Electronics 1987:84–91.

[30] Nath S, DiMarco JP, Haines DE. Basic aspects of radiofrequency catheter ablation. J Cardiovasc Electrophysiol 1994;5:863–76.

[31] Fink B, Schneider T, Braunstein S, et al. Holmium: YAG laser-induced aseptic bone necroses of the femoral condyle. Arthroscopy 1996;12(2):217–23.

[32] Owens BD, Stickles BJ, Balikian P, et al. Prospective analysis of radiofrequency versus mechanical debridement of isolated patellar chondral lesions. Arthroscopy 2002;18(2):151–5.

[33] Stein DT, Ricciardi CA, Viehe T. The effectiveness of the use of electrocautery with chondroplasty in treating chondromalacic lesions: a randomized prospective study. Arthroscopy 2002;18(2):190–3.

[34] Vangsness Jr CT, Mitchell III W, Nimni M, et al. Collagen shortening. An experimental approach with heat. Clin Orthop 1997;337:267–71.

ELSEVIER
SAUNDERS

Orthop Clin N Am 36 (2005) 433 – 446

ORTHOPEDIC
CLINICS
OF NORTH AMERICA

Treatment of Full-thickness Chondral Defects with Autologous Chondrocyte Implantation

Scott D. Gillogly, MD*, Thomas H. Myers, MD

Atlanta Sports Medicine and Orthopaedic Center, 3200 Downwood Circle, Suite 500, Atlanta, GA 30327, USA

With the introduction of new treatment methods for cartilage repair over the past 10 to 15 years, a corresponding interest has developed in gaining a better understanding of the scope of the clinical problem and classification of cartilage injuries. Although an understanding of the natural history of cartilage injuries in the knee remains elusive, this interest has nonetheless elucidated the scope, complexity, and diversity of cartilage injuries. Certainly all cartilage defects do not produce the same degree of clinical symptoms, progress at the same rate toward osteoarthritis, or require the same uniform treatment. Consideration must be given to the size, depth of involvement, location, and number of the defects. Additionally, individual patient parameters such as age, body mass, activity demands, and perhaps most importantly the condition of the remainder of the knee all influence treatment decision making. The investigators have learned that failure to address any copathologies of the knee, such as mechanical malalignment, ligamentous instability, or deficient meniscal function, will expose any cartilage repair process to a continued overload environment and often doom the clinical outcome. Therefore, not all cartilaginous injuries require the same treatment, and treatment must be tailored to the individual patient and cartilage lesion.

As with any new and innovative treatment methods, there have been constant refinements in technique, indications, and clinical expectations for these recent advances in cartilage repair. The new techniques of cellular repair with autologous chondrocyte implantation, and tissue transfer with osteochondral autografts and allografts, have continued to evolve with further scrutiny toward optimizing the results from these treatment methods. Although no treatment option is universally ideal for all full-thickness cartilage defects, the goal remains a repair that can restore the normal surface congruity of the joint, control the patients' symptoms, maintain the characteristics to withstand the intra-articular forces of the knee over time, and prevent the progression of focal chondral injuries to diffuse osteoarthritis [1]. These newer treatment methods continue to be evaluated for their consistency and reproducibility of outcomes, durability of repair, and cost-effectiveness [2].

The technique of autologous chondrocyte implantation (ACI), first reported by Brittberg and colleagues [3] in 1994, has found a major role in the treatment of large full-thickness chondral injuries. In this technique, a small biopsy of healthy chondral tissue is obtained arthroscopically when the lesion is identified and then undergoes in vitro chondrocyte cell culture, returning a 12-fold increase in the number of cells available for implantation into the defect at the second stage of the procedure. The principle behind using autologous chondrocytes is to produce a repair tissue that more closely resembles the morphologic characteristics of hyaline cartilage and is therefore better able to restore the durability and natural function of the knee joint [3,4]. As experience around the world has grown and the durability of the repair tissue has been demonstrated with good clinical outcomes seen beyond a decade postoperatively, indications and confidence in the

---

* Corresponding author.
E-mail address: sdg14@mindspring.com
(S.D. Gillogly).

technique have expanded to include treatments for more complex knee pathologies in combination with large articular cartilage defects [4–6].

Indications for autologous chondrocyte implantation

The predominant indication for ACI is symptomatic, large full-thickness chondral lesions located on the femoral condyles or the trochlear groove, including osteochondritis dissecans (OCD) in patients from adolescent age to the fifties. It is also important for patients to be willing and able to comply with the postoperative rehabilitation protocol. ACI is not indicated as a treatment option for severe osteoarthritis, as defined by the presence of bipolar bone on bone lesions. If a large lesion is present on the reciprocal surface (kissing lesions) with exposed bone, greater than a grade III chondromalacia, the opposing surface is typically not suitable for this technique [3,7–9]. This fact is particularly true when secondary bony deformity exists as a result of the arthritic process. There are, however, exceptions to this general rule, namely trochlea and patellar defects or femoral condyle lesions with small tibial lesions in the milieu of an absent meniscus. In these special cases, which usually occur in younger patients, options exist for resurfacing these defects and correcting the underlying knee pathologies.

Results of treating isolated chondral injuries of the patella and tibia with ACI have not been as consistent as those of treating the femoral condyles and trochlea [3]. However, with better understanding of the importance of patellar alignment, the results of patellar ACI have improved. The indications for ACI treatment of the tibia include a traumatic substantial-sized defect in a younger patient. Degenerative lesions on the tibia are rarely indicated for this technique of chondral resurfacing. ACI is contraindicated in active inflammatory arthritis or infection. Prerequisites for a successful outcome with ACI also include appropriate bony alignment; ligamentous stability; meniscal function; adequate motion and muscle strength; and compliance, in addition to a focal chondral injury in a knee without significant bony arthritic changes.

Patient selection and preoperative evaluation

As experience with biologic resurfacing of cartilage injuries has grown, it has become apparent that the assessment of the condition of the overall knee is as important as the assessment of the chondral defect itself. The presence of coexisting knee pathology, such as ongoing ligamentous instability, bony malalignment, or complete meniscal deficiency, will prevent an environment conducive for cartilage repair [5,7]. Any abnormalities in these factors must be addressed before or concomitant with treatment of the cartilage defect with ACI. Failure to recognize and treat these coexisting factors will result in poorer patient outcomes or complete failure of the resurfacing procedure.

A thorough history provides the first step in assessing patient suitability for ACI. Additionally, it is important to confirm that symptoms are coming from the chondral injury. This confirmation is particularly relevant to patients who have undergone prior repair techniques, such as marrow stimulation for the cartilage defect. Perhaps the repair has been adequate and further symptoms are from incomplete rehabilitation of the patellofemoral joint with corresponding anterior knee complaints and not symptoms from a previously treated femoral condyle lesion. Typically patients who have condyle lesions will have pain with weight-bearing or increased loading circumstances; complaints of catching or partial locking; recurrent swelling; and point tenderness in the area of the defect. The presence of a trochlear or patellar lesion will have similar findings, but will include aggravation of pain associated with stairs, getting in and out of a chair or car, and anterior knee pain. Patellar subluxation symptoms are often also present. Additional information is often available on patients who have known articular cartilage lesions through previous operative reports, previous studies, and intraoperative video photographs of prior procedures. Taking advantage of any available information will help in determining the suitability of the defect for ACI.

Physical examination includes motion assessment, basic ligamentous examination, provocative meniscal tests, and patellar tracking tests. Additionally, careful palpation of each compartment and accessible chondral surface will give further clues as to potential sources of the patients' complaints. Although examination gives a good indication of involved compartment and the presence or absence of other knee pathology, additional testing with appropriate radiographs and MRI will be necessary. These studies will aid in confirming the results of the clinical examination.

To adequately evaluate a patient for ACI, it is essential that weight-bearing anterior-posterior (AP) and 45° posterior-anterior (PA) and patellar alignment radiographs be obtained [5,10,11]. These radiographs allow initial assessment of the alignment of the tibiofemoral and patellofemoral portions of the joint and give an indication of any underlying bone involvement associated with the defect from OCD or a traumatic osteochondral defect. A long leg limb alignment view to assess the mechanical axis is used to definitively determine the potential need for realignment osteotomy (Fig. 1). MRI can then be used to assess the ligament and meniscal status and to define the degree of subchondral bone involvement [12]. Increased signal and edema in the subchondral bone of a chronic nature may indicate persistent overload of the involved compartment, making realignment a more likely adjunct to cartilage resurfacing. Bone loss of greater than 7 to 8 mm in depth requires bone grafting before or at the time of cell implantation.

The most definitive step in assessing the suitability of a chondral lesion for ACI comes at the time of arthroscopic evaluation. The size, location, and depth of the defect; the status of the surrounding articular cartilage and underlying bone; and the status of the opposing chondral surfaces are all evaluated. Containment of the defect is also assessed. In other

words, does the bordering rim of healthy articular cartilage fully surround the defect or do the margins of the defect fade into the intercondylar notch or perimeter of the condyle or trochlea? This assessment is important as it may indicate that special techniques will be necessary to secure the periosteal patch to hold the autologous chondrocytes during implantation. When assessing the cartilage status, it must be determined whether the joint will be improved with resurfacing of the defect or if the degenerative process is too advanced diffusely within the joint with multiple involved bipolar surfaces, in which case ACI or any other biologic resurfacing procedure will be inadequate in improving the patient's symptoms. The ideal chondral lesion to repair with ACI is a full-thickness defect surrounded by healthy, normal-appearing cartilage in an otherwise healthy knee. Any deviation from the ideal may require specific variations in technique or concomitant procedures to address additional pathology. Generally, the defects treated by this technique are larger than 2 cm^2; the average size in the investigators' series has been well over 5 cm^2 [3,5,7]. Arthroscopic assessment also gives an opportunity for examination under anesthesia to confirm ligament stability and

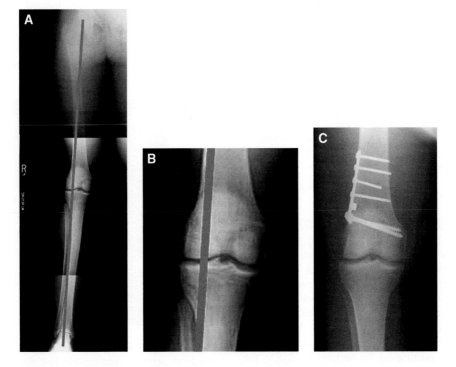

Fig. 1. (A,B) Long limb alignment film demonstrating the mechanical axis shifted to the lateral compartment, well lateral to the lateral tibial spine in a patient who has a lateral femoral condyle full-thickness chondral defect. (C) Realignment with lateral opening distal femoral osteotomy performed concomitantly with ACI treatment of the lateral femoral condyle defect.

allows evaluation of the meniscal function and patellofemoral tracking.

Surgical technique

Chondral biopsy

The surgical technique for ACI requires two
stages: one to obtain a chondral biopsy for growing
the autologous chondrocytes and another for implantation of the cells within the chondral defect.
The essential steps include an initial chondral biopsy
for autologous chondrocyte cell culture obtained at
the time of arthroscopic assessment. The biopsy is
obtained from the superior peripheral edges of the
lateral or medial femoral condyles superior to the
sulcus terminalis or from the inner edge of the intercondylar notch. The investigators have found an
arthroscopic gouge to be the easiest tool to use to
obtain several small slivers of healthy chondral tissue for the biopsy. The total volume needed is roughly
equivalent to the size if a pencil eraser and is typically
three or four slivers measuring about 5 × 10 mm,
with the thickness of the healthy articular cartilage.
After the biopsy fragments are removed from the
knee with arthroscopic graspers, they are placed in
the biopsy medium/shipping vial in sterile fashion
and forwarded for cell culture. The ACI procedure
is then performed at a second stage consisting of
arthrotomy, defect preparation, periosteal procurement, fixation of the periosteal tissue, creation of a
watertight seal with fibrin glue, implantation of
the chondrocytes, and wound closure [3,5–9]. The
time between the biopsy and the implantation
can be as short as 3 to 6 weeks or can wait months
until the optimal time as determined by the patient
and surgeon.

Surgical exposure

The amount of exposure necessary for the implant
procedure arthrotomy is determined by the size and
location of the defect. A midline incision is generally
recommended, followed by a medial or lateral parapatellar arthrotomy, exposing the corresponding
chondral injury. As with any surgical procedure,
it is essential that the full extent of the defect
is exposed, facilitating all the technical aspects of
the implantation. Inadequate exposure can lead to the
incomplete securing of the periosteal patch to the
defect, possibly resulting in cell leakage or graft
delamination. Multiple, complex, or hard-to-reach
chondral injuries often require a larger midline

incision with a medial parapatellar arthrotomy and
eversion of the patella. When performing a concomitant patellar realignment procedure, the investigators
have detached the tubercle and turned the tubercle
and patella proximally, giving wide exposure to the
knee (Fig. 2). The tubercle is then reattached with
cortical screws in the realigned position after the
cell implantation.

Defect debridement

During debridement of the defect, all damaged
and unhealthy appearing cartilage and fibrocartilage
is removed using small curettes, leaving exposed
subchondral bone with a rim of stable cartilage
around the circumference of the defect. Failure to
debride the calcified zone of cartilage inhibits the
integration of the repair tissue to the subchondral
bone [13]. Any thinned, fissured, or damaged surrounding cartilage needs to be debrided to an edge,
leaving healthy firm articular cartilage. This technique provides a stable nonmobile edge to affix the
periosteal patch and decreases the risk for micro-
motion of the patch during rehabilitation with
incumbent increased risk for graft delamination or
periosteal hypertrophy [14]. During debridement, the
subchondral bone should not be violated. Penetration
of the subchondral bone leading to bleeding potentially introduces stem cells and fibroblasts into the
defect that can compromise the quality of the repair
tissue. If bleeding in the defect is encountered,

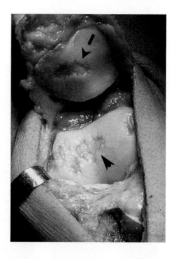

Fig. 2. The tibial tubercle has been detached and turned
proximally, allowing excellent exposure for ACI of the
trochlea and patellar defects (*arrows*). Anteromedialization
of the tibial tubercle is typically combined with ACI of the
trochlea or patella.

hemostasis should be obtained for any bleeding bone. Techniques to control any bleeding bone include using compression over the area with epinephrine-soaked neuro-patties with a dilute 1 to 1000 epinephrine and saline solution. Thrombin spray or temporary gel-foam may also be used. Fibrin glue may be applied to the bleeding area and then compressed with a neuro-patty. In refractory punctate bleeding from the bone, electrocautery with a needle-point Bovie set at a low setting of 5 to 8 W can be the final step for controlling bleeding. In some cases, internal or intralesional intra-articular osteophytes in the subchondral bone may be encountered during debridement of the defect. These osteophytes can be the result of penetration of the subchondral bone either from injury or prior surgical procedures, such as drilling or microfracture, and are more common in chronic lesions These bony prominences can be addressed by gently tapping them back into the subchondral bone plate with a smooth, noncorrugated bone tamp [5,15]. Attempts to excise or curette the osteophytes will otherwise lead to excessive bleeding within the defect. The goal of adequate debridement of the defect is to have a dry defect with clean subchondral bone and a healthy surrounding cartilage border at the periphery. Defect dimensions can then be measured using a sterile ruler to determine the size of the defect. The best method for obtaining the correct size for the periosteal graft is to create a template from the sterile paper that comes with surgical gloves. A template can be made by placing a slightly larger-sized piece of the paper over the defect and outlining the defect with a marking pen. The template is then cut around the pen markings, oversizing by 1 to 1.5 mm around the circumference. The purpose of slightly oversizing the template is to account for the fact that the periosteum has a tendency to shrink slightly after harvest.

Periosteal harvest

The next step is to obtain a periosteal graft to be transferred to the defect and secured to contain the cells. The periosteum harvest is from the proximal medial tibia, two fingerbreadths distal to the pes anserinus and medial collateral ligament insertion on the subcutaneous border. A separate incision is made just anterior to the posterior border of the tibia. The periosteum is easily accessible at this location, using blunt dissection down through the overlying subcutaneous fat. All fat and fascia layers should be removed from the periosteum using sharp and blunt dissection with a moist sponge. Leaving the thin fascia layer or fat on the periosteum is one of the most common

mistakes made with harvesting the periosteal graft [16]. The template is then placed over the exposed periosteum, a 15 blade used to sharply demarcate the periosteal graft, and a sharp curved periosteal elevator used to gently dissect the periosteum from the bone. Smooth forceps can be used on the leading edge of the periosteum to provide countertraction for subperiosteal dissection. Obesity, inactivity, smoking, and increased age may lead to atrophy of the periosteum [15,17]. In the event that the proximal medial tibia periosteum is thin and inadequate, an alternate site for periosteal procurement is the distal femur. Rather than use the distal femoral periosteum just proximal to medial and lateral femoral condyle articular surfaces, the investigators have found the periosteum on the metaphyseal flare of the femur to be closer to typical tibial periosteum and not as overly thick as the more distal femoral periosteum. This tissue can easily be exposed by a limited subvastus approach, lifting the vastus medialis anteriorly to expose this second source of periosteum. Regardless of which periosteal harvest site is used, the final graft should be a clean contiguous layer without holes or excessive fat or fascia on its outer surface. Although the medial femoral metaphysis serves as a good backup source, usually the proximal tibia serves as the best and most consistent source for periosteal graft harvest.

Securing periosteal graft

The periosteal graft is then aligned over the defect in the orientation matching the template, with the cambium layer of the periosteum facing the defect. The periosteum is next sutured to the cartilage rim with multiple interrupted 6-0 Vicryl sutures spaced every 2 to 3 mm. The knots should be tied on the periosteal side, not on the surface of the cartilage, thus minimizing any friction or toggling that could cause loosening of the knots. Securing the periosteum works best if several sutures are placed superiorly and then inferiorly to ensure proper tension on the graft, creating a drumlike effect. The contour of the site should be recreated and the graft should fully cover the defect and cover medial to lateral. Typically as the "corners" are secured, it becomes apparent that there is some redundancy of the graft that can be trimmed with sharp scissors to keep appropriate tension on the graft. Having several different needle choices for these small sutures is helpful because of the variation in cartilage thickness present in most knees. Although a smaller needle with a shorter radius of curvature works best around thick normal cartilage, a thin needle with a greater radius of curvature allows a longer pass through thinner cartilage and therefore holds the suture better than a shorter pass. Once all the sutures are in place with only a small opening remaining, the watertight integrity of the graft can be tested using an 18-gauge catheter attached to a saline-filled tuberculin syringe placed deep to the periosteum through the small opening. By slowly filling the defect with saline, any leakage can easily be seen around the perimeter of the repair site and any additional sutures can be placed as necessary. Next the suture line at the periosteal graft–defect interface is sealed using any of the commercial preparations of fibrin glue available in most operating rooms to assure a watertight seal of the chondral edges and the periosteum by acting as a rapidly setting sealant.

Implantation of autologous chondrocytes

The autologous chondrocytes are then sterilely aspirated from their shipping vial into a sterile tuberculin syringe using an 18-gauge plastic angiocatheter and injected under the periosteal graft into the defect. Each vial contains about 10 to 12 million chondrocytes and provides more than adequate cells for defects up to 10 cm^2. The injection site is then closed with one or two additional sutures and sealed with fibrin glue (Fig. 3). At this point the ACI is complete and all retractors are removed from the knee. The knee should be brought into full extension, ensuring that there is no contact with any opposing surface during the maneuver. Any further wound hemostasis or irrigation is then performed, making sure that there is no inadvertent contact with the graft and no deep suction is used. Any concomitant procedures should be completed before implanting

the chondrocytes, as no additional manipulation of the joint should follow the implantation. The arthrotomy and wound are then closed in a layered fashion and a soft sterile dressing and knee immobilizer applied to the knee. A drain is not routinely used because of the potential for damage to the graft by contact or from the suction effect of the drain. The postoperative course and rehabilitation are discussed later.

Complex defects

Uncontained chondral lesions

In cases where the defect is not fully contained by a rim of healthy cartilage, special techniques may be necessary to secure the periosteum and still establish a watertight seal. Locations where defects often involve at least one uncontained border include those extending to the intercondylar notch such as OCD defects of the medial femoral condyle, the proximal margin of the patella, the lateral margin of trochlear defects from patellar dislocations, and the posterior lateral femoral condyle in lateral OCD. If a synovial fringe of tissue exists and is still well attached to the margin of the bone, the periosteum can be attached securely to the synovium. More frequently, there is no appropriate soft tissue for fixation and only bone surface remains at the margin. In these cases, absorbable microanchors loaded with 5-0 absorbable suture and the smallest free needle available work well in securing the periosteum directly to the bone in the uncontained portion of the defect. Usually three

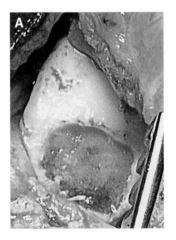 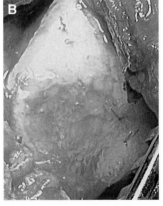

Fig. 3. (*A*) This lateral femoral condyle defect has been debrided down to subchondral bone, ensuring the removal of the calcified cartilage layer. The edges of the surrounding cartilage are distinct and the lesion is well contained. (*B*) Final appearance of the defect after the periosteum has been secured, sealed with fibrin glue, and the cells injected under the periosteum.

to four anchors are used and should be placed first, and then each sequential suture is brought through the periosteum in a vertical mattress fashion. The periosteum tends to bunch up when using this method, so the investigators tend to oversize the periosteum a little more for uncontained lesions. The investigators have never seen an anchor pull out, either intraoperatively or postoperative. Following securing the periosteum at the uncontained portion of the defect, the remaining periosteum is sutured and the suture line sealed with fibrin glue.

Multiple chondral lesions

Despite more extensive involvement in knees with multiple chondral lesions, good to excellent outcomes are still possible with ACI [18]. Provided the remaining knee is free of significant bony arthritic changes, and coexisting knee pathologic conditions are corrected, excellent outcomes with ACI, comparable to smaller lesions, can be achieved. The main factors to consider when undertaking multiple lesions treated with ACI are (1) extensile exposure, (2) whether multiple vials of cells will be available, and (3) whether it is possible to obtain sufficient periosteum. Generally, it is feasible to obtain two typical-sized grafts from the usual proximal tibia site. Both templates should be placed on the periosteum to achieve the best orientation and use of available periosteum before cutting the grafts (Fig. 4). The investigators have used the contralateral tibia in several cases where there was previous surgery at the tibia and

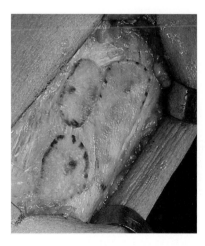

Fig. 4. Multiple periosteal grafts can be harvested from the proximal tibia through a separate incision on the posteromedial margin of the proximal tibia just distal to the pes tendons. Note how the templates are laid out before cutting the grafts to ensure maximization of all available periosteum.

there is concern about adequate periosteum. The distal femur should also be used when necessary for multiple defects.

Massive chondral lesions

A massive chondral defect is defined as a lesion greater than 8 cm^2. The investigators have used ACI on defects over 20 cm^2 with outcomes similar to more usual-sized defects. Provided that the knee is non-arthritic and coexisting pathologic conditions are addressed, excellent outcomes can be expected when treating massive chondral defects with ACI. One significant difference, however, is the time required for the maturing repair tissue to heal. It will take longer for maturation and therefore the rehabilitation process is controlled accordingly. The investigators have also used an unloader brace during the first 6 months postoperative in cases where an osteotomy was not necessary. Special planning is again required for periosteum harvest similar to the techniques used for multiple defects. These massive-sized chondral lesions are also more likely to have uncontained cartilage borders, and the technique of securing the periosteum with microanchors is frequently used. As a general rule, one vial of cells contains approximately 10 to 12 million autologous cultured chondrocytes, and should be used for each 8 to 10 cm^2 of a defect. Therefore, at least two vials of cells need be available for massive defects. Additionally, to ensure uniform disbursement of the cells, the investigators will inject the cells with one vial of cells at the midpoint of the defect and another at the superior aspect of the defect, closing each injection site sequentially with additional sutures and fibrin glue.

Copathology and concomitant procedures

Good results with autologous chondrocyte implantation, like any method of cartilage repair, should not be expected if coexisting knee pathology is not addressed.

As a greater understanding of the clinical presentation of articular cartilage lesions has developed, it has become apparent that there are typically multiple factors that contribute to intra-articular knee problems. It is therefore predictable that there will often be coexisting knee pathologic conditions accompanying large chondral defects. Regardless of whether or not any coexisting knee pathologic conditions contributed to or occurred simultaneous with the chondral injury, the presence of continued knee pathologic conditions is clearly detrimental to

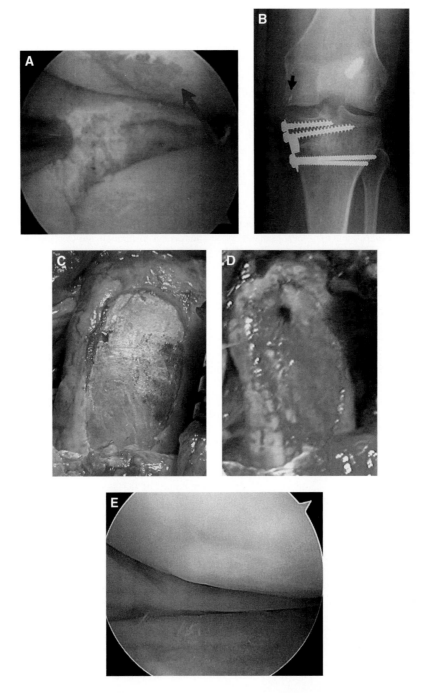

Fig. 5. (*A*) Arthroscopic view of medial compartment in a 39-year-old woman who had chronic anterior cruciate ligament (ACL) deficiency after failed reconstruction. Note the absent medial meniscus and medial femoral condyle full-thickness chondral defect. The patient underwent multiple procedures in two stages to include revision ACL reconstruction with patellar tendon allograft, medial opening high tibial osteotomy, medial meniscal allograft transplantation, and ACI of the medial femoral condyle massive full-thickness chondral defect that was partially uncontained. (*B*) Radiograph showing the medial opening high tibial osteotomy (HTO), ACL fixation, and metallic microsuture anchors for the uncontained portion of the ACI. (*C,D*) Medial femoral condyle (MFC) defect at the time of ACI. (*E*) Final arthroscopic view 24 months after completion of all stages of this complex knee reconstruction showing intact medial meniscus transplantation and excellent resurfacing of the MFC defect with ACI.

restoring articular cartilage function and durability. The maturation of the repair tissue can be severely altered or inhibited in a compromised environment. When ACI is used to repair articular cartilage defects in the presence of coexisting pathologic conditions, it is essential that the intra-articular environment of the knee be restored to as close to normal as is possible. As discussed later, aggressive evaluation and diagnosis needs to be accompanied by definitive treatment of the coexisting knee pathologic conditions. This treatment can be accomplished as a staged procedure or concomitant with ACI. Biomechanical malalignment, maltracking, meniscal deficiency, and ligamentous insufficiency are examples of an altered intra-articular environment that can lead to shear stresses, excessive friction, and abnormal compressive loads across the injured chondral surface [5,19]. Therefore, it is critical that associated knee pathologic conditions, including mechanical malalignment (of the tibiofemoral joint and the patellofemoral articulation), ligamentous instability, and meniscal deficiency, be corrected before or in conjunction with the cells being implanted (Fig. 5). Another issue to be assessed is the degree of underlying bone damage to the subchondral bone, especially in OCD lesions or traumatic osteochondral injuries [5,6,10,20]. Failure to recognize coexistent knee pathologic conditions before autologous chondrocyte implantation will dramatically reduce the chances of a good outcome [4,5,18].

When deficiencies are present in any of these areas, treatment needs to be planned to maximize the recovery of the patient while still addressing the various copathologies. Many factors, such as the degree or severity of the deficiency, total number of problems, age of the patient, and the patient's ability to comply with postoperative restrictions, go into determining the best approach to each patient situation. In the investigators' experience, performing only one additional procedure at the same time as the ACI is preferred. This practice would include performing an anterior cruciate ligament (ACL) reconstruction or osteotomy, or meniscal transplantation or anteromedialization of the tibial tubercle in addition to the ACI [5,20]. However, when more extensive coexisting knee pathologic conditions exist whereby three or more definitive reconstructive procedures may be indicated, staging seems more prudent. This practice is intended to cut down on the effect of cumulative potential complications [1,21]. Although there is no absolute answer as to when to include a concomitant procedure versus staging, the investigators have not found an increased risk for complications when combining ACI with one additional

procedure. Of the initial 156 patients undergoing ACI in one study, 86 patients (55%) underwent a concomitant procedure, including anteromedialization of the tibial tubercle (60 patients), ACL reconstruction (16 patients), HTO (8 patients), and meniscal transplantation (8 patients). An additional 17 patients (11%) underwent a staged procedure, either bone grafting of an osteochondral defect (9 patients) or HTO (8 patients) [5].

Tibiofemoral malalignment

Biomechanical malalignment is typically addressed at the time of ACI. The type and location of the osteotomy depends on the type and degree of deformity. The traditional recommendations for osteotomy correction of knee malalignment calls for overcorrecting the deformity to shift the mechanical axis into the opposite compartment [22,23]. Although that practice may be appropriate for treatment of osteoarthrosis, the purpose of osteotomy associated with cartilage resurfacing is to decrease the forces in the overloaded compartment and balance the forces across the joint. As many of these patients with full-thickness chondral defects are younger in age, they would not tolerate an overcorrection that they would view as a deformity. The investigators have found it more appropriate to aim at shifting the mechanical axis to the 50% mark in the middle of the tibial spines. The investigators have increasingly used medial opening wedge high tibial osteotomy, either with plate fixation or external fixation with medial hemicallotasis for overload of the medial compartment. For overload of the lateral compartment, either a lateral-opening tibial HTO with fibular osteotomy is used, or for bigger corrections or bone deformity on the lateral femoral condyle from OCD, a lateral-opening distal femoral osteotomy with a locking plate is used. The investigators favor a closing-wedge tibia osteotomy in patients who are smokers, whereas the medial hemicallotasis technique is better-suited for staged ACI procedures. If the osteotomy is performed concomitantly with ACI, the suturing of the periosteum and implantation of the cells are completed after the osteotomy.

Ligamentous insufficiency

Persistent ligamentous insufficiency produces excessive shear forces across the chondral surfaces in the knee. Even subtle laxity or giving way of the knee can result in unacceptable forces across the maturing cells, resulting in damage to the maturing repair tissue produced by autologous chondrocyte implantation. ACL tears have been the most common ligamentous injury the investigators have seen with full-thickness chondral injuries [5]. Posterior cruciate ligament reconstruction also can accompany ACI. Typically performed concomitantly, ACL reconstruction should be completed before proceeding with ACI. The ligament reconstruction should be performed in standard fashion with whatever technique and graft are desired by the surgeon and patient. Arthroscopic ACL reconstruction should be completed before proceeding with the arthrotomy for the ACI. In cases where exposure may be a problem, such as very posterior condylar or any tibial defect, it may be beneficial to wait for final fixation of the tibial side of the ACL graft until the ACI procedure is completed. No specific accommodation to the ACL rehabilitation protocols are needed because the ACI rehabilitation program is more limiting and is the overriding guidance postoperatively.

Meniscal deficiency

Determining when a partial meniscectomy leads to a loss of meniscal function equivalent to a total meniscectomy is not easy. The posterior third of the menisci are more important than the anterior third in terms of function. Also, the peripheral fibers of the menisci providing the hoop-stress function are particularly essential [24]. Volume of lost meniscus alone is not the only criterion in determining deficient meniscal function, as even a small-appearing radial tear of the meniscus can dramatically diminish the function. Meniscus transplantation should be considered in knees that have had a total meniscectomy performed in the same compartment as the chondral injury [20,25,26]. A meniscal allograft will help to reduce the concentrated forces in the involved compartment and help protect the newly formed repair tissue [20,26]. The exact indications are still unclear. The investigators tend to favor meniscal transplantation in younger patients and adolescents who have complete absent menisci, and certainly if early tibial articular wear is present. The older patients who have longstanding meniscectomy may be better-served with osteotomy. It is interesting to note that of all the patients reported from the extensive Swedish series, with its high percentage of good and excellent results at long-term follow-up, no patients underwent meniscal transplantation, as that procedure is unavailable in that country [4]. One could logically conclude that meniscal transplantation is the least-essential component to a successful clinical outcome. Once again, the decision of whether to perform meniscal transplantation as a staged procedure or concomitantly with ACI depends on surgeon and patient preference. If there is any question, staging the two procedures seems more prudent. When performed concomitantly, the meniscal transplantation should be performed first using the surgeon's standard technique, followed by completion of the ACI. Clinical experience in this area is limited; however, Gersoff [20] has preliminarily reported on ten patients who have had concomitant meniscal allograft transplantation and ACI with 80% success at 2-year follow-up.

Patellofemoral malalignment

Abnormal patellar tracking is not only the likely source of the patellar or trochlear injuries but would also preclude an environment conducive for the maturation of the implanted chondrocytes into the ideal hyaline-like repair tissue. In addition to the concerns of lateral maltracking of the patella, the concept of decreasing the patellofemoral contact forces is also desirable. Depending on the degree of lateral maltracking, the amount of medialization can be adjusted accordingly. The anteromedialization of the tibial tubercle as described by Fulkerson [27] offers the option of adjusting the degree of medialization while still elevating the tubercle anteriorly. In some cases without lateral maltracking, anterior transfer of the tibial tubercle alone may be sufficient to reduce the contact pressure of the patellofemoral articulation.

In most cases of patellar or trochlear chondral injuries, a distal patellar realignment procedure should be performed in combination with ACI. In the investigators' series of 92 patella or trochlea ACI procedures, 88 out of 94 patients (94%) underwent concomitant anteromedialization of the tibial tubercle. Although the patellar realignment can be performed with the initial arthroscopy, the investigators have found it more prudent to almost always combine the distal realignment with the ACI for patellar or trochlear defects, allowing the tubercle to be turned up proximally and giving extensile exposure as noted earlier. Regardless of whether the surgeon elects a concomitant realignment or a staged procedure, patellofemoral alignment, tracking, and load distribution need to be optimized at the time of ACI, providing the chondrocytes the optimal environment for maturation [10].

Bone deficiency

One situation that routinely requires staging is the treatment of bone deficiency. In cases where the bony deficiency of the defect exceeds 7 to 8 mm in depth, a separate staged bone grafting procedure is performed. With further experience, the initial technique of open bone grafting has been replaced with an arthroscopic technique. After arthroscopic debridement of any necrotic bone in the base of the defect, autologous bone is harvested from the proximal tibia or distal femur through a cortical window and then a core harvest instrument from an osteochondral graft set. The harvest sites are backfilled with off-the-shelf bone graft plugs. The autologous bone is then interspersed with allograft paste and inserted into the debrided bony defect through an 8- to 10-mm cannula, impacted, and sealed with fibrin glue. Fluid inflow to the knee is turned off during the arthroscopic grafting, impaction, and fibrin glue application. The ACI procedure can then be performed at least 4 to 6 months later after the bone graft has incorporated. Bone grafting allows restoration of the level of the subchondral bone and gives a healthy base for the chondrocytes to attach and grow (Fig. 6) [16]. Additionally, it minimizes the amount of hyaline-like repair tissue that must be regenerated in the defect, speeding up ultimate maturation. Staged bone grafting is usually performed at the time of arthroscopic evaluation and chondral biopsy.

Another newer technique is the so-called sandwich bone grafting technique that allows single-stage bone grafting of a bony defect in combination with ACI. In this procedure, the defect is exposed with an arthrotomy as described earlier and the base of the defect debrided of necrotic bone. Bone graft is then obtained either from the iliac crest or from the distal

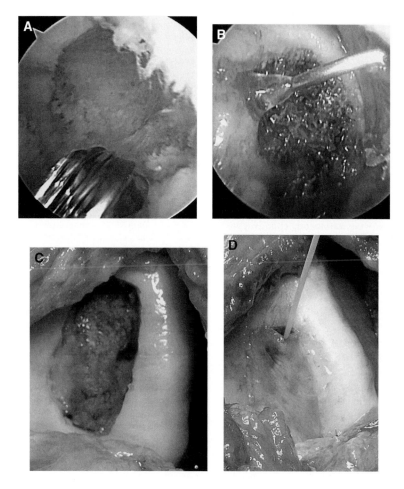

Fig. 6. OCD defect of the lateral femoral condyle with bone loss greater than 8 mm treated with staged arthroscopic bone grafting. (*A*) Arthroscopic debridement of the necrotic bone in the base of the defect. (*B*) Arthroscopic autologous cancellous bone graft impacted into the defect and sealed with fibrin glue after the inflow is turned off. (*C*) During ACI after 6 months to allow healing of the graft, the defect shows healed bone in the base up to the level of the subchondral bone. (*D*) Periosteum in place and cells being injected under the periosteal graft.

femur or proximal tibia as described earlier. The investigators have favored taking local bone from around the knee and backfilling the donor site, rather than expose the patient to the morbidity of an iliac crest harvest. The bone graft is then impacted into the defect up to the level of the subchondral bone. Using sterile glove paper, a template is then made of the size of the defect's base and a first periosteal graft is harvested corresponding to the template. This first periosteal graft is then placed in the defect with the cambium side up toward the joint and secured with sutures either into the base of the rim of articular cartilage or with absorbable suture anchors into the bone. Fibrin glue then seals the deep perimeter separating the blood and marrow elements from the defect. Another template is then made for the size of the articular cartilage defect identical to the routine ACI procedure. This template is then used to harvest a second periosteal graft that is secured to the chondral surface with the cambium side down toward the defect, again in an identical fashion to the basic ACI procedure. The cells are then injected below the outer layer of periosteum, thus "sandwiching" the cells between the two layers of periosteum with their cambium layers facing the cells. The bone graft then consolidates concurrent to the chondrocytes maturing. This procedure is technically demanding. Advancement of weight-bearing and loading exercises are typically delayed after this procedure.

Rehabilitation following autologous chondrocyte implantation

Rehabilitation following ACI is based on the maturation process of the chondrocytes, the size of the defect, and the location of the defect [5–7,9]. The concept of a slow gradual maturation of the repair tissue is crucial to understanding the rehabilitation following ACI [7]. The biologic nature of the hyaline-like repair tissue must be protected and stimulated to allow the maturation and remodeling of the tissue. Premature overload of the repair tissue will increase the likelihood of failure. There are three basic phases associated with this healing process: the proliferative phase, the matrix production phase, and the maturation phase. Each successive phase can accommodate greater degrees of load, allowing the addition of sequential weight-bearing, exercise, and impact. Fully mature repair tissue that might take 12 to 24 months in the maturation process shows stiffness very close to the surrounding articular cartilage [9]. During the initial phase of rehabilitation, the critical elements are motion (to help with cellular orientation and the prevention of adhesions), protection of the graft from mechanical overload, and strengthening exercises to allow for a functional gait. Continuous passive motion is started 6 to 12 hours after surgery. Initial touch weight-bearing is usually progressed to full weight-bearing after 4 to 6 weeks postoperatively. Addition of further exercises should be based on the size, location, and amount of containment of the lesion by normal surrounding cartilage. The knee is gradually loaded with increased strengthening exercises after 3 months and various impact-loading activities after 6 months. The patella and trochlea are protected from open-chain exercises and shear loading for at least the first 3 months. Adhering to these principles during the repair maturation continuum will provide an optimum environment for the tissue to grow and mature [5,7,9]. The addition of concomitant procedures does not require any change to the rehabilitation principles, as the ACI program remains the rate-limiting step while still satisfying the rehabilitation principles of early motion and progressive joint loading.

Clinical results

ACI has been performed for over a decade in the United States and Europe and almost 2 decades in Sweden. Peterson and colleagues [9] have reported a retrospective analysis on the first 100 patients treated with ACI, with follow-up ranging between 2 to 9 years. Out of 25 patients who had isolated femoral condyle chondral lesions, 23 (92%) had successful outcomes, whereas 16 out of 18 (89%) patients who had osteochondral defects had good to excellent results. Multiple rating scales, including the Modified Cincinnati, Tegner, and Lysholm scores were used to assess the clinical and functional outcomes. Additionally, they reported a 96% durability of good to excellent results initially at 2-year follow-up, with 30 of 31 patients maintaining those results at 7.5-year follow-up [9]. The overall clinical outcomes remained constant (80% good to excellent results at 2 years, and 78% at 7.5 years) and second-look arthroscopies did not show signs of tissue breakdown. Additionally, experience has grown rapidly in the United States and Europe, further documenting and defining the clinical applicability of this technique [5,9,14,18,28–32].

Other international centers with at least 2-year follow-up have reported comparable outcomes to the Swedish series. Bahuard [28] reported good to excellent clinical outcomes with military personnel in 84% of 24 patients, showing that most of the patients were able to return to military duty following ACI. Further series from Norway and the United Kingdom show similar clinical results and also show histologic data on biopsies, with 75% of the specimens showing hyaline-like repair tissue [14,30]. Bentley and colleagues [29] reported on a prospective randomized study comparing ACI and mosaicplasty that found 88% excellent and good results with ACI versus 69% in the mosaicplasty group at 19-months follow-up. One-year second-look arthroscopies showed 82% excellent and good repairs in the ACI group versus only 34% in the mosaicplasty group. Horas and associates [33] reported on 40 patients randomly assigned to ACI or mosaicplasty for chondral injuries. At 2 years, both group had improved pain, although the ACI group lagged behind the mosaicplasty group on Lysholm scores. Histologically, the ACI group showed fibrocartilage superficially and hyaline-like repair tissue closer to the subchondral bone. Knutsen and colleagues [34] reported a randomized controlled study of 40 patients treated with microfracture and 40 patients treated with ACI at four centers with 2-year follow-up. Both methods showed acceptable outcomes at this early follow-up and there were no significant differences on macroscopic appearance or histologic findings.

Minas and Chiu [18] reported results on 235 patients treated with autologous chondrocyte implantation, showing an 87% success rate over a 6-year period. Most of their patients had complex lesions with coexistent knee pathology or were salvage patients who had early degenerative changes such as osteophytes or some joint-space narrowing. Minas and colleagues [6,18] have also noted that salvage patients who have early degenerative changes do not obtain as high activity scores after ACI as compared to ACI patients without early degenerative changes; however, these salvage patients have the highest patient-satisfaction ratings, perhaps because they were starting at very difficult baseline levels.

The author's clinical results with the initial 112 patients treated with ACI have shown a 91% good to excellent success rate over a 5-year period [5]. Of the 54 patients who had a 2-year or longer follow-up, significant improvements from the baseline scores were noted in each of the assessment tools used (Modified Cincinnati Rating Scale, Knee Society Clinical Rating, and Sports Score), with a consistent progression over time. The average clinician and patient evaluations of overall knee function showed significant improvement from baseline, and showed an improvement on an annual basis. The baseline scores for clinician and patients were scores of 3.9. The 24-month follow-up showed improvement in

knee function with a significant increase ($P < .001$) in average score to 8.3 and 7.9. At 36, 48, and 60 months, the clinician and patient scores continued to show improvement over baseline without decline in function over time. Additional subgroup analysis has showed no statistical difference in outcomes for gender, size of the defect, location of the defect on the femur, isolated versus multiple defects, or ACI with concomitant procedure or alone. There was, however, a statistical difference, with better results associated with lesions treated within 1 year from injury or onset of symptoms than in chronic defects present for greater than 1 year [1,21].

The Cartilage Registry Report, an international multicenter observational assessment of patients treated with ACI, has revealed that 78% of all defects treated with ACI had improvement by patient assessment, whereas 81% of isolated femoral condyle defects had improved. Clinician evaluations have shown a 79% improvement for all lesions and an 85% improvement in femoral condyle lesions. The most common adverse event reported with ACI is intra-articular adhesions (2%). The next most common adverse events include detachment/delamination less than 1% [31].

Summary

ACI is a reproducible treatment option for large full-thickness symptomatic chondral injuries with appropriate knowledge of technique and patient selection. It provides a cellular repair that offers a high percentage of good to excellent clinical results over a long follow-up period. ACL is applicable over a wide range of chondral injuries from simple to more complex lesions. For successful cartilage repair, it is essential that the intra-articular environment be as close to normal as possible. Coexisting knee pathology must be aggressively treated. ACI does have a prolonged postoperative rehabilitation course necessitated by the biologic nature of the repair, and patients must be able to comply with the rehabilitation and temporary restrictions required for a successful outcome.

The next generation of cellular repair for cartilage defects is optimistic. Newer techniques, such as embedding the autologous cells in a biologic matrix, augmenting their maturation with growth factors, and other forms of cell regulation, are some of the options currently being investigated. Matrix ACI implantation without the need for a periosteal patch has already been performed at some centers in Europe. With further basic science and clinical research, the reproducibility, ease of surgical delivery of the autologous cells, and results should only improve.

References

[1] Gillogly SD. Treatment of large full-thickness chondral defects of the knee with autologous chondrocyte implantation. Arthroscopy 2003;19(Suppl 10):S147–53.

[2] Minas T. Chondrocyte implantation in the repair of chondral lesions of the knee: economics and quality of life. Am J Orthop 1998;27:739–44.

[3] Brittberg M, Lindahl A, Nilsson A, et al. Treatment of deep cartilage defects in the knee with autologous chondrocyte transplantation. N Engl J Med 1994;331:889–95.

[4] Peterson L, Lindahl A, Brittberg M, et al. Autologous chondrocyte transplantation: biomechanics and long-term durability. Am J Sports Med 2002;30(1):2–12.

[5] Gillogly SD. Autologous chondrocyte implantation: complex defects and concomitant procedures. Oper Tech Sports Med 2002;10:120–8.

[6] Minas T, Peterson L. Advanced techniques in autologous chondrocyte transplantation. Clin Sports Med 1999;18(1):13–44.

[7] Gillogly SD, Voight M, Blackburn T. Treatment of articular cartilage defects of the knee with autologous chondrocyte implantation. J Orthop Sports Phys Ther 1998;28(4):241–51.

[8] Minas T. Autologous cultured chondrocyte implantation in the repair of focal chondral lesions of the knee: clinical indications and operative technique. J Sports Traumatol Rel Res 1998;20:90–102.

[9] Peterson L, Minas T, Brittberg M, et al. Two to nine year outcomes after autologous chondrocyte transplantation of the knee. Clin Orthop Relat Res 2000;374:212–34.

[10] Hamby TS, Gillogly SD, Peterson L. Treatment of patellofemoral articular cartilage injuries with autologous chondrocyte implantation. Oper Tech Sports Med 2002;10:129–35.

[11] Rosenberg TD, Paulos LE, Parker RD, et al. The forty-five-degree posteroanterior flexion weight-bearing radiograph of the knee. J Bone Joint Surg Am 1988;70:1479–83.

[12] Recht MP, Resnick D. Magnetic resonance imaging of articular cartilage: an overview. Top Magn Reson Imaging 1998;9:328–36.

[13] Breinan HA, Minas T, Hsu H, et al. Effect of cultured autologous chondrocytes on repair of chondral defects in a canine model. J Bone Joint Surg Am 1997;79:1439–51.

[14] Richardson J, Caterson B, Evans E, et al. Repair of human articular cartilage after implantation of autologous chondrocytes. J Bone Joint Surg Br 1999;81:1064–8.

[15] Peterson L. Cartilage cell transplantation. In: Malek MM, editor. Knee surgery—complications, pitfalls, and salvage. New York: Springer-Verlag; 2001. p. 440–9.

[16] Brittberg M. Autologous chondrocyte transplantation. Clin Orthop Relat Res 1999;367(Suppl):S147–55.

[17] O'Driscoll SW. Articular cartilage regeneration using periosteum. Clin Orthop Relat Res 1999;367S:186–203.

[18] Minas T, Chiu R. Autologous chondrocyte implantation. Am J Knee Surg 2000;13(1):41–50.

[19] Minas T. Nonarthoplasty management of knee arthritis in the young individual. Curr Opin Orthop 1998;9:46–52.

[20] Gersoff W. Combined meniscal allograft transplantation and autologous chondrocyte implantation. Oper Tech Sports Med 2002;10:1165–7.

[21] Gillogly SD. Autologous chondrocyte implantation. Sports Med Arthroscopy Rev 2003;11(4):272–84.

[22] Hernigou P, Medevielle D, Debeyre J, et al. Proximal tibial osteotomy for osteoarthritis with varus deformity. A ten to thirteen-year follow-up study. J Bone Joint Surg Am 1987;69:332–54.

[23] Slocum DB, Larson RL, James SL, et al. High tibial osteotomy. Clin Orthop Relat Res 1974;104:239–43.

[24] Grood ES. Meniscal function. Adv Orthop Surg 1984;7:193–7.

[25] Veltri DM, Warren RF, Wickiewicz TL, et al. Current status of allograft meniscal transplantation. Clin Orthop Relat Res 1994;303:44–55.

[26] Verdonk PCM, Demurie A, Almqvist F, et al. Transplantation of viable meniscal allograft. J Bone Joint Surg Am 2005;87:715–24.

[27] Fulkerson JP. Anteromedialization of the tibial tuberosity for patellofemoral malalignment. Clin Orthop Relat Res 1983;177:176–81.

[28] Bahuard J, Maitrot R, Bouvet R, et al. Implantation of autologous chondrocytes for cartilaginous lesions in young patients. A study of 24 cases. Chirurgie 1998;123(6):568–71.

[29] Bentley G, Biant LC, Carrington RW, et al. A prospective, randomised comparison of autologous chondrocyte implantation versus mosaicplasty for osteochondral defects in the knee. J Bone Joint Surg Br 2003;85:223–30.

[30] Haugegaard M, Lundsgaard C, Vibe-Hansen H. Treatment of cartilage defects with autologous chondrocyte implantation—preliminary results. Acta Orthop Scand 1998;2(69):11.

[31] Mandelbaum B, Browne J, Fu F, et al. Current concepts on articular cartilage lesions of the knee. Am J Sports Med 1998;26:853–61.

[32] Peterson L. International experience with autologous chondrocyte transplantation. In: Insall JN, Scott WN, editors. Surgery of the knee. 3rd edition. New York: Churchill Livingstone; 2000. p. 341–56.

[33] Horas U, Pelinkovic D, Herr G, et al. Autologous chondrocyte implantation and osteochondral cylinder transplantation in cartilage repair of the knee joint. J Bone Joint Surg Am 2003;85:185–92.

[34] Knutsen G, Engebretsen L, Ludvigsen TC, et al. Autologous chondrocyte implantation compared with microfracture in the knee. A randomized trial. J Bone Joint Surg Am 2004;86:455–64.

ELSEVIER
SAUNDERS

Orthop Clin N Am 36 (2005) 447–458

ORTHOPEDIC
CLINICS
OF NORTH AMERICA

Arthroscopic Osteochondral Autografting

David A. Coons, DO, F. Alan Barber, MD*

Plano Orthopedic and Sports Medicine Center, 5228 West Plano Parkway, Plano, TX 75093, USA

Arthroscopic osteochondral autografting is one of many techniques to treat chondral damage. Osteochondral transplantation transfers a plug of healthy articular cartilage, tidemark, and subchondral bone into matching zones at a defect site. The advantages of this procedure include the repair of a defect by hyaline articular cartilage (not fibrocartilage) and the maintenance of the articular height and shape. Arthroscopic osteochondral autografting is a single-stage procedure with minimal costs and can be performed on an outpatient basis. An entirely arthroscopic transplantation can be technically challenging, and larger lesions are difficult to fully treat because of limited availability of donor material.

Indications and contraindications

The indications for arthroscopic osteochondral autografting are single, full-thickness lesions between 1 and 2.5 cm in diameter (Fig. 1) [1–4]. Larger defects (greater than 2.5 cm in diameter) are associated with poorer results (Fig. 2) [5,6]. In addition, this technique is generally limited to lesions with subchondral bone loss not exceeding 6 mm in depth (Fig. 3) [1]. Autologous osteochondral transplantation is not recommended for bipolar lesions (corresponding type IV tibial damage), knees with multiple type IV lesions, or patients who have unstable or malaligned knees. Diminished benefits can be expected in patients who are older than 35 years, and some authors do not recommend this procedure for patients who are older than 50 years [7]. Other contraindications include a history of joint

infection, intraarticular fracture, rheumatoid arthritis, and generalized degenerative arthritis (Fig. 4) [1,7]. Meniscal tears and ligament instability are not absolute contraindications, but these conditions should be corrected at the time of autografting [2,8–10]. Osteochondral autografting is most commonly performed on the femoral condyles, although autografting of tibial plateau, trochlea, and patella lesions has been reported [1,3,11–13].

Instrumentation

The chondral osseous replacement (COR) system (DePuy Mitek, Marlborough, Massachusetts) allows for the harvesting of precisely sized osteochondral plugs and their transplantation to precisely drilled defects. Several other systems exist to accomplish this procedure, including the Osteochondral Autologous Transfer System (Arthrex, Naples, Florida), Mosaicplasty system (Smith & Nephew, Andover, Massachusetts), and soft delivery system (SDS; Sulzer Orthopedics, Austin, Texas). The distinctive differences for the COR system are the cutter tooth in the harvester that allows for a precise depth of cut (Fig. 5) and the use of a drill for lesion preparation (Fig. 6). Using a drill for lesion preparation makes it easier to orient the recipient hole vertically to the adjacent articular cartilage surface, and the control afforded by the precise harvest cut allows the surgeon to prepare the recipient site accurately before donor harvest.

Technique

A thorough arthroscopic diagnostic knee evaluation should be performed first. When a localized, full

---

* Corresponding author.

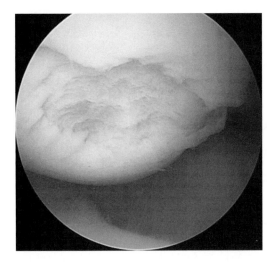

Fig. 1. The indications for arthroscopic osteochondral autografting are single, full-thickness lesions between 1 and 2.5 cm in diameter.

thickness osteochondral defect in encountered, it is important to visualize all areas of the knee, including the posterior recess and beneath the menisci to identify and remove any mobile chondral fragments (Fig. 7). Arthroscopic transplantation is possible for most lesions; however, large and very posterior lesions may require extreme knee flexion to achieve an angle perpendicular to the articular cartilage. This angle is sometimes more readily achieved by an arthrotomy. A spinal needle can be used to determine the best angle for portal creation, ensuring a perpendicular approach to the harvest and defect

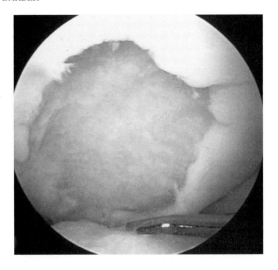

Fig. 3. Arthroscopic osteochondral autograft transplantation is generally limited to lesions with subchondral bone loss not exceeding 6 mm in depth.

sites. There are five steps to arthroscopic osteochondral autografting: (1) evaluation and preparation of the lesion, (2) determining the number of grafts, (3) graft harvest, (4) preparation of the insertion site, and (4) graft delivery.

Evaluate and prepare the lesion

The knee and lesion should be carefully evaluated to verify that the inclusion criteria are met and that

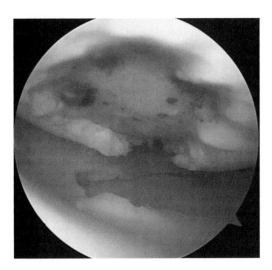

Fig. 2. Larger defects (greater than 2.5 cm in diameter) are associated with poorer results.

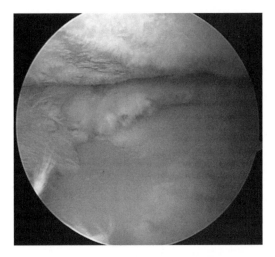

Fig. 4. Contraindications include joint infection, intra-articular fracture, rheumatoid arthritis, and generalized degenerative arthritis.

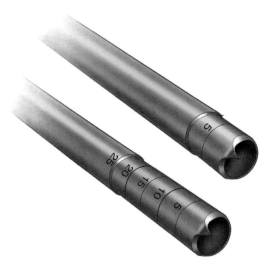

Fig. 5. The COR harvester cutter tooth allows for a precise depth of cut. (*Courtesy of* DePuy Mitek, Norwood, MA; with permission.)

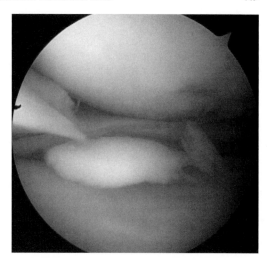

Fig. 7. It is important to visualize all areas of the knee, including the posterior recess and beneath the menisci, to identify and remove any mobile chondral fragments.

there are no contraindications to the procedure. The defect is prepared by removing any loose articular cartilage debris and freshening the edges of the lesion with a curette (Fig. 8) or an arthroscopic knife to create perpendicular chondral walls. The subchondral bone should be cleared of any residual articular cartilage, but generalized bone bleeding should be avoided. For planning purposes, the initial transplanted plug should be placed immediately adjacent to the articular cartilage in the most anterior area of the defect.

Determine the number of grafts

Once the margins have been defined, the number of grafts required is determined by using the probe (Fig. 9) or the harvester to measure the defect size and depth, and to determine which configuration of plugs best fits the defect. The depth of the lesion can be estimated with the COR system by using a probe or the measurement etchings on the side of the harvester as a guide. In general, a series of 6-mm di-

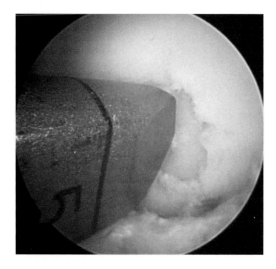

Fig. 6. A drill is used to create the recipient sites in the lesion.

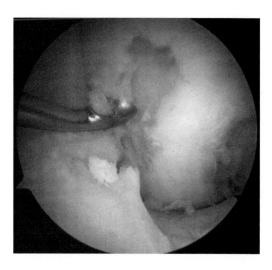

Fig. 8. Defect preparation includes removing loose articular cartilage debris and creating vertical lesion edges with a curette.

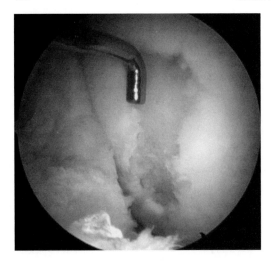

Fig. 9. The number of grafts required is determined by using the probe or harvester.

ameter grafts can be transplanted and arranged arthroscopically to fill the defect. Larger plug harvesters are available but they often require a mini-arthrotomy for harvest and are more likely to result in encroachment of the higher weight-bearing areas at the donor sites.

The depth of the defect should also be analyzed. Most lesions do not have significant bone loss. In these cases, the standard 8-mm harvester depth is sufficient to fill the defect. However, some lesions (especially those of osteochondritis dissecans) have significant bone loss that should be addressed. This situation may be dealt with by bone grafting the lesion at one procedure and returning to perform the transplantation later, or by using the variable depth harvester and placing grafts that have cancellous sections standing above the crater base (Fig. 10).

An assessment of the donor site and recipient site articular cartilage contours is also important to match the chondral surfaces as optimally as possible during transplantation. For larger defects, the use of multiple plugs is effective in recreating the original contour of the condyles. Although the use of smaller plugs allows for greater contouring, this benefit is offset by decreased strength and stability of the transplanted plugs and an increased number of steps.

Graft harvest

Once the number of plugs to be obtained is determined, the harvester is inserted into the dispos-

able cutter. The retropatellar fat pad should be debrided before instrument insertion to improve visualization and avoid soft tissue entrapment. A blunt plunger is placed in the harvester tube to minimize soft tissue capture while inserting the instrument into the knee. The harvester should be positioned perpendicular to the desired harvest site and the blunt plunger replaced with the anvil to provide an impaction surface and to avoid fluid loss through the harvester tube. The common donor sites for this harvest are the superior lateral intercondylar notch and the lateral trochlear ridge above the linea terminalis.

Using a mallet, tap the anvil impaction surface (continuing to hold the harvester perpendicular to the articular cartilage in all planes) until the harvester's offset lip or the desired depth mark (when using a variable depth harvester) reaches the articular cartilage surface. Overly aggressive impaction of the variable depth harvester may result in abnormally long plugs. A unique feature of the COR system is the cutter tooth on the harvester blade (see Fig. 5). This cutting tooth underscores the cancellous bone at the distal end of the harvester tube and allows for a precise depth cut. The T-handle of the harvester is rotated two full revolutions and the plug is removed by gently twisting the T-handle while withdrawing (Fig. 11). Care should be taken to avoid any toggling or rocking of the harvester as it is removed to avoid widening the donor site any more than necessary. Next, the harvester tube is disassembled from the

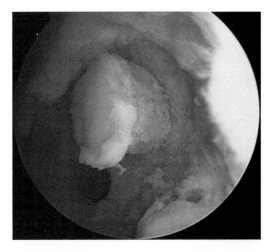

Fig. 10. The variable depth harvester may be used to address lesions with significant bone loss by placing grafts with cancellous sections standing above the crater base.

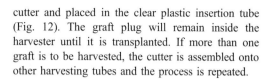

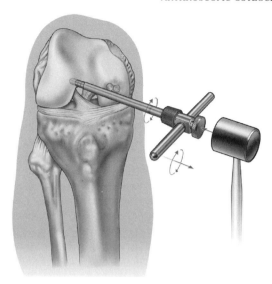

Fig. 11. After impaction to the depth stop or appropriate laser depth line, the T-handle of the harvester is rotated two full revolutions and the plug is removed by gently twisting the T-handle while withdrawing. (*Courtesy of* DePuy Mitek, Norwood, MA; with permission.)

cutter and placed in the clear plastic insertion tube (Fig. 12). The graft plug will remain inside the harvester until it is transplanted. If more than one graft is to be harvested, the cutter is assembled onto other harvesting tubes and the process is repeated.

Insertion site preparation

The recipient sites are drilled with the COR drill bit corresponding to the harvester that was used (Fig. 13). The recipient site drill is slightly smaller than the harvester to allow a secure press-fit of the transplanted plug. Drilling should be done under direct arthroscopic visualization, keeping the drill oriented perpendicular to the adjacent articular cartilage surface. The projecting tooth on the tip of the drill allows for a precise placement by creating a starter hole and avoids the drill "walking away" from the desired location. The drill should be advanced to the offset articular cartilage depth stop when using the standard harvester, or to the appropriate laser line when using the variable depth harvester. In cases of

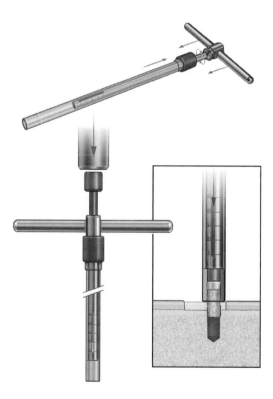

Fig. 12. The harvester tube is placed in the clear plastic insertion tube (*Courtesy of* DePuy Mitek, Norwood, MA; with permission.)

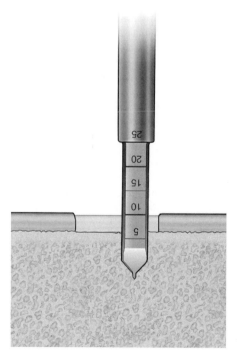

Fig. 13. The recipient sites are drilled with the COR drill bit corresponding to the harvester that was used. (*Courtesy of* DePuy Mitek, Norwood, MA; with permission.)

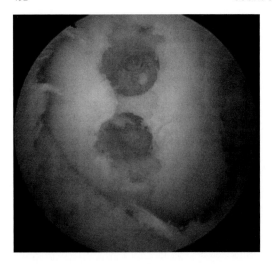

Fig. 14. All recipient holes can be drilled at once and should be separated by a 1- to 2-mm bone bridge.

subchondral bone loss, the depth may be underdrilled to restore the contour and height of the articular surface (see Fig. 10). All holes can be drilled at once or drilled sequentially after filling the individual recipient sites. Care should be taken to separate the recipient sites by 1 to 2 mm to maintain a bone bridge (Fig. 14) and to keep the drill holes parallel to avoid recipient site convergence.

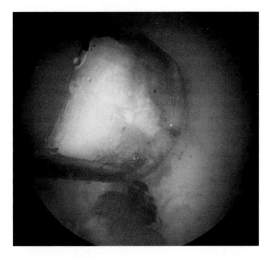

Fig. 15. The clear end of the delivery system is placed at the recipient site, perpendicular to the articular surface, and rotated to align the donor articular cartilage correctly with the recipient articular cartilage surface.

Graft delivery

The plastic plunger of the harvester-delivery system is gently tapped with the mallet to advance the osteochondral plug into the clear portion at the distal end of the delivery guide. Additional careful tapping will advance the plug 1 to 2 mm out of the end of the delivery guide to aid in aligning the plug into the recipient site.

Once the insertion sites are prepared, the loaded harvester clear-plastic delivery guide system is inserted into the knee. The portal chosen may need to be slightly enlarged to permit this passage. The clear end of the delivery system with the slightly projecting graft tip is placed at the outlet of the drill recipient site and, while the inserter is held perpendicular to the adjacent articular cartilage, rotated to orient the articular cartilage surface of the graft to an optimal alignment with the recipient articular cartilage surface (Fig. 15). The graft is then implanted by gently tapping until the articular cartilage is flush with the articular cartilage of the adjacent femoral

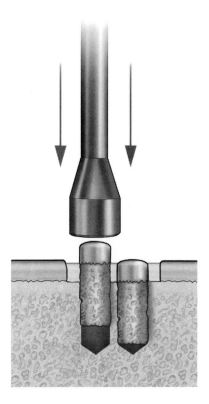

Fig. 16. A tamp or the plastic plunger may be used to fine-tune this graft placement. (*Courtesy of* DePuy Mitek, Norwood, MA; with permission.)

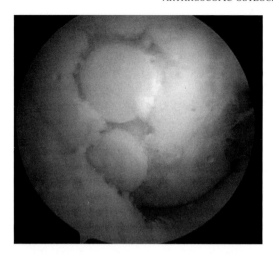

Fig. 17. The process is repeated until the repair is complete.

condyle. A tamp or the plastic plunger may be used to fine-tune this graft placement (Fig. 16). Additional plugs are placed using the same technique (Fig. 17).

Harvest sites

The superior medial femoral condyle, the superior lateral femoral condyle above the linea terminalis, and the superior lateral intercondylar notch have been proposed as graft harvest sites (see Fig. 11). Contact pressures, curvature matches, and cartilage thicknesses have been studied to identify optimal harvest sites [14–17]. Ideally, grafts should be harvested from minimal weight-bearing areas to decrease morbidity. In general, contact pressures are lower in the intercondylar notch and medial trochlea [14,18]. However, only a small area is available for harvest before areas of increased contact pressure are encountered. Although contact pressures are higher in the lateral trochlea, they decrease as the harvest site is moved distally. Harvesting just anterior to the linea terminalis has been recommended when using the lateral trochlea [16,18]. The superior lateral intercondylar notch is commonly obliterated in anterior cruciate ligament reconstruction without obvious morbidity and seems to provide adequate tissue with low morbidity risk.

An analysis of cartilage thickness and curvature using stereophotogrammetric examination found the distal medial trochlea and intercondylar notch to be superior donor sites based on the low donor site involvement in load-bearing [14]. In contrast, topographic matching using laser techniques found the lateral and medial trochlea curvatures to better match the recipient sites on the femoral condyles when compared with the intercondylar notch [15]. Other investigators have recommended the anterior portion of the lateral trochlea based on cartilage thickness and curvature [4,16]. The saddle-shaped portion of the anterior intercondylar notch better matched the recipient sites of the central trochlea [14]. In addition, the articular cartilage was thinnest at the linea terminalis (less than 1 mm) and thickest in the central trochlear [16].

Graft stability

Graft stability is directly influenced by the diameter and length of the plug [19]. Longer grafts were harder to pull out than shorter grafts. Specifically, the pullout failure loads of 10-mm-long grafts were significantly lower (47 N) than 15- or 20-mm-long grafts (mean, 93 and 110 N) using 11-mm diameter grafts in a porcine model. Additionally, grafts that were reinserted after an initial pull-out test had a failure strength of less than half that of the original insertion strength (mean, 93 N versus 44 N). In this same test, larger diameter grafts were harder to pull out than smaller grafts. Failure loads of 8-mm diameter grafts (mean, 41 N) were significantly lower than those of 11-mm diameter grafts (mean, 92 N) of the same length [19]. The method of harvesting was also shown to make a difference. Levering of the plug harvester during the graft harvest significantly decreased the subsequent press-fit stability when compared with simple turning of the harvester [19].

Harvest techniques

The location of the graft harvest influences the ability to obtain perpendicular osteochondral grafts. Plugs harvested from the lateral trochlear ridge were statistically more perpendicular than the plugs harvested from the intercondylar notch. However, no statistically significant difference was noted between open and arthroscopic harvesting techniques [20]. These findings may be clinically insignificant, as implantation angles up to 10° have been reported without complications [1].

Whether the grafts are harvested manually or with power is another factor. Power trephine harvesting has been shown to decrease chondrocyte viability when compared with manual punch harvesting [21]. Power harvesting was technically more difficult and resulted in more gross and light microscopic damage to the osteochondral grafts. Manual harvesting was not found to affect the stiffness, surface irregularity, and thickness of the cartilage of the plugs at time zero [22].

Graft implantation

Oversizing the graft appears to be essential to preserving the histologic properties of the chondral cap and is probably related to increased stability. Grafts that were oversized by 1 mm showed no significant histologic changes, whereas grafts that were harvested and replaced in the same holes showed an increase in cartilage thickness and cell density. Round and polygonal hypertrophic clusters of chondrocytes with cytoplasmic vacuoles were observed [23,24].

Although ideal, placement of the graft flush to the adjacent articular cartilage to decrease contact stresses is not often achieved. Placement within 1 mm of the articular surface was found in only one third of the patients evaluated postoperatively by MRI [17]. The peak contact pressures at the defect site were found to increase by 20% once the recipient hole was created. These contact pressures dropped back to normal when the inserted plugs were placed flush to the adjacent articular cartilage. Plug elevation as little as 0.5 mm increases contact pressures almost 50% compared with flush plugs [25,26]. In an animal model, although grafts left 2-mm proud repositioned themselves after weight-bearing, perigraft fissuring, fibroplasia, and subchondral cavitations were the result [27]. Depressed plugs were found to have elevated pressures of about 10% [25].

In another study, specimens that were placed in a flush position demonstrated minimal thickening or changes in the histologic architecture of the articular cartilage. In contrast, those specimens countersunk 1 mm demonstrated significant cartilage thickening (54.7% increase). Chondrocyte hyperplasia, tidemark advancement, and vascular invasion occurred at the chondro-osseous junction of these grafts while the surface remained smooth. In grafts countersunk 2 mm, cartilage necrosis and fibrous overgrowth were observed [28].

Histology

A major advantage of osteochondral transplantation is the restoration of hyaline cartilage instead of less-durable hyaline-like cartilage or fibrocartilage [10]. Biopsies from second-look arthroscopic cases confirm the survival of the hyaline cartilage in the

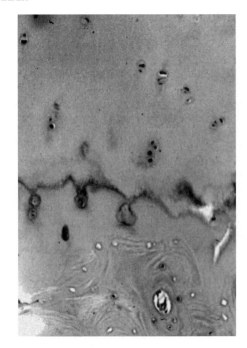

Fig. 18. Biopsies from second-look arthroscopies confirm the survival of the hyaline cartilage in the transplanted osteochondral plugs.

transplanted osteochondral plugs (Fig. 18) [3,4,10, 12,29]. Histologically, no evidence of cartilage repair at the host/graft junction is seen; rather, islands of transplanted hyaline cartilage are joined with a fibrocartilage "grout." The underlying cancellous bone shows normal bony bridging between native peripheral tissue and grafts [28,29]. Cellular viability in autogenous osteochondral plugs is not statistically different from controls at 6 months after surgery. The indentation stiffness of the transferred plug and the contralateral donor site were similar. Both were much stiffer than normal cartilage, including the surrounding condylar cartilage [30].

Donor sites

Clinically, the donor sites for 4- and 6-mm grafts have been observed to fill without grafting and cover with a fibrocartilagenous scar on second-look arthroscopies [3,10,29]. However, graft-site morbidity, including excessive postoperative bleeding and mild to moderate pain, has been reported with an incidence of 3% of patients who were undergoing mosaicplasty using 4- and 6-mm plugs [10]. Most symptoms (95%) resolved within 6 weeks, but persistent pain was reported. Harvesting larger plugs that encroach on weight-bearing surfaces and excessive plug harvesting seem to be the most likely causes [10,15,31].

Jackson and colleagues [32] recently studied the fate of full-thickness osteochondral defects in a sheep model. Untreated, full-thickness 6 × 6-mm defects on the femoral condyle did not heal. A "zone of influence" was found on the surrounding cartilage, leading to thinning and flattening of the articular surface. A progressive increase in the size of the defect was observed with the formation of a large cavitary lesion and the collapse of the surrounding subchondral bone and articular cartilage into the periphery of the defect. The investigators suggest that the size of the defect may reach a critical diameter at which increased compressive forces lead to mechanical overloading of surrounding bone and cartilage. Messner and Gillquist [33] have reviewed cartilage repair and refer to this detrimental loading adjacent to defects as "edge stress." In their report, 12 of 31 patients who had a single unipolar lesion of at least 10 mm in diameter had radiographic joint-space reduction of more than 50% at a 14-year follow-up.

In a human cadaver study, increased stress concentrations around the rims of condylar defects 10 mm in diameter and greater were seen. In lesions 8 mm in diameter or less, the meniscus was able to effectively absorb increases in pressure [31,34]. It is likely that the harvest site location in addition to the diameter and depth of the harvested plug are independent risk factors leading to harvest site morbidity. Cur-

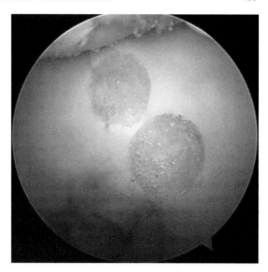

Fig. 20. These donor sites were backfilled with the TruFit prosthesis (OsteoBiologics, San Antonio; TX), which is currently undergoing a multicenter evaluation of its use to reduce donor site morbidity.

rently, the critical defect size, depth, and ratio of these factors that lead to increased morbidity in humans are not known. These studies give insight as to what mechanisms might play a role in harvest site morbidity. They certainly justify the treatment of unipolar lesions 10 mm in diameter. These data also lead to the question that if a lesion 10 mm in diameter is a reasonable candidate for treatment, how reasonable is it to create a lesion 10 mm in diameter to obtain a graft for such a repair?

Grafting the harvest defects with material from the lesion [35] or a synthetic material (backfilling) may decrease donor site morbidity by preventing defect sidewall erosion and providing a substrate that encourages bony ingrowth and surface repair. One such synthetic device is made with polylactide-co-glycolide, polyglycolide, and calcium sulfate (Fig. 19). This bone graft substitute implant can be used to backfill harvest sites and is currently undergoing a multicenter evaluation of its use in reducing donor site morbidity (Fig. 20). These plugs have been studied in knee defects in an animal model [36]. Observations at various intervals up to 1 year after implantation demonstrated no significant cratering or osteophytes. These observations suggest a stable articulation with the adjacent articular cartilage. A histologic analysis of these sites confirmed bony ingrowth and surface repair with predominantly hyaline cartilage in the animal model [36]. Another study reported fibrocartilage surface repair using various materials to fill defects [37]. Back-

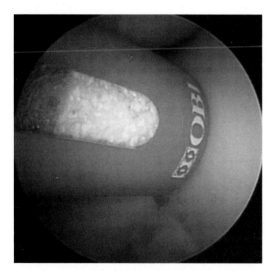

Fig. 19. Grafting the harvest defects with a synthetic material (backfilling) may decrease donor site morbidity by preventing defect sidewall erosion and providing a substrate that encourages bony ingrowth and surface repair.

filling defects may decrease excessive bleeding and reduce donor site morbidity.

Allograft

Clinical outcome studies using allograft osteochondral plug grafts have not been reported. Chondrocyte viability in press-fit glycerol-preserved osteochondral allografts was recently compared with fresh autografts. Microscopic and histologic examination demonstrated a positive effect from load-bearing on the osteochondral allografts. Grafts transplanted into load-bearing sites had higher chondrocyte viability (77% ± 17% SD) than those transplanted into non–load-bearing sites (25% ± 2%). A positive effect from load-bearing was not seen in autografts, however. In addition, load-bearing allografts demonstrated histologic scoring closer to that of autografts and adjacent cartilage, all of which fared significantly better than non–load-bearing allografts. Load-bearing allografts had more fibrocartilage than autografts or adjacent cartilage, but less fibrocartilage than non–load-bearing allografts. Autografts and allografts had non-significant increases in metabolism compared with adjacent cartilage as measured by sulfate-uptake [38]. The use of allograft material may play a role in minimizing donor site morbidity in the future, but significantly increased costs and a minimal risk for disease transmission remain concerns.

Results

Condylar lesions typically have excellent clinical outcomes. A review of 10 years of experience reported good to excellent results in 92% [7]. Many other authors have reported a similar outcome at 24, 42, and 45 months follow-up [1,3,12]. The authors have previously reported that the average Lysholm scores improved from 33 and 44 preoperatively to 81 and 88 postoperatively [1,3]. In IKDC assessment, 87% of patients reported their knees to be normal or nearly normal at 45 months follow-up [3]. No difference in contour or appearance was seen on relook arthroscopies [29,39]. Postoperative MRI evaluation revealed that articular surface congruency had been restored in 92% of patients, although an abnormal subchondral marrow signal was seen in 75% even after 4 years [3].

The results from tibial lesions and patellar and trochlear mosaicplasty were not as consistent. Good to excellent results were reported in 87% of those treated with tibial resurfacing compared with 79%

treated with patellar and trochlear resurfacing [14]. Ma and colleagues [12] reported fair results in two patients who had lesions on the tibial surface, whereas Nakagawa and colleagues [13] reported good results in a patient who had bilateral trochlea mosaicplasties.

Traumatic chondral lesions treated with osteochondral transplantation resulted in good or excellent results in more than 80% of patients [5,12,40]. The best results were obtained with isolated chondral lesions and patients who required fewer grafts. Osteochondral transplantation has also been used to successfully treat osteochondritis dissecans [35] and osteonecrosis of the femur [9]. The underlying diagnosis, including osteonecrosis, osteochondritis dissecans, and traumatic cartilage defects, did not affect the clinical outcome. However, lesions larger than 6 cm^2 were associated with increasing fibrous tissue formation, fissuring between the grafts and host tissues, and poor results [40]. Increasing patient age also corresponded with poorer outcomes. If the patients were younger than 30 years, there was a 90% return to normal pain-free activity, whereas only 23% of the patients older than 30 years returned to normal pain-free activity [10].

Finally, comparisons have been made between various cartilage treatment options. Autologous osteochondral transplantation has been compared directly to autologous chondrocyte implantation (ACI). Biopsies at intervals up to 24 months after surgery noted the formation of hyaline cartilage in autologous osteochondral transplants, whereas fibrocartilage was observed in the ACI patients [41]. Autologous osteochondral transplants have been also been compared in a multicenter, comparative, randomized study of marrow stimulation procedures, such as microfracture, Pridie drilling, and abrasion arthroplasty. Results at 3 to 6 years follow-up showed durable improvement in the clinical outcome with autologous osteochondral transplantation, in contrast to the marrow stimulation procedures. The marrow stimulation resulted in fibrocartilage formation and diminished clinical results, especially after 3 years postoperatively [11].

Summary

Arthroscopic osteochondral autografting is indicated for unipolar, full-thickness articular cartilage lesions between 1 and 2.5 cm in diameter. A stable, properly aligned knee is important to a good outcome. This procedure should not be performed in the presence of generalized osteoarthritis. Arthroscopic osteochondral autografting allows the restoration of hyaline articular cartilage with zonal matching of the graft. It is cost-effective, can usually be performed on an outpatient basis, and results in durable resurfacing with excellent long-term results.

References

[1] Barber FA, Chow JC. New frontiers in articular cartilage injury. Arthroscopy 2003;19(10):142–65.

[2] Bobic V. Arthroscopic osteochondral autograft transplantation in anterior cruciate ligament reconstruction: a preliminary clinical study. Knee Surg Sports Traumatol Arthrosc 1996;3(4):262–4.

[3] Chow JC, Hantes ME, Houle JB, et al. Arthroscopic autogenous osteochondral transplantation for treating knee cartilage defects: a 2- to 5-year follow-up study. Arthroscopy 2004;20(7):681–90.

[4] Hangody L, Rathonyi GK, Duska Z, et al. Autologous osteochondral mosaicplasty. Surgical technique. J Bone Joint Surg Am 2004;86(Suppl 1):65–72.

[5] Delcogliano A, Caporaso A, Menghi A, et al. Results of autologous osteochondral grafts in chondral lesions of the knee. Minerva Chir 2002;57(3):273–81.

[6] Hangody L, Kish G, Karpati Z, et al. Mosaicplasty for the treatment of articular cartilage defects: application in clinical practice. Orthopedics 1998;21:751–6.

[7] Hangody L, Fules P. Autologous osteochondral mosaicplasty for the treatment of full-thickness defects of weight-bearing joints: ten years of experimental and clinical experience. J Bone Joint Surg Am 2003; 85(Suppl 2):25–32.

[8] Gross AE. Cartilage resurfacing: filling defects. J Arthroplasty 2003;18(3 Suppl 1):14–7.

[9] Kotani A, Ishii Y, Sasaki S. Autogenous osteochondral grafts for osteonecrosis of the femoral condyle. J Orthop Surg (Hong Kong) 2003;11(2):117–22.

[10] Hangody L, Kish G, Kárpáti Z. Arthroscopic autogenous osteochondral mosaicplasty – a multicentric, comparative, prospective study. Index Traumat Sport 1998; 5:3–9.

[11] Hangody L, Feczko P, Bartha L, et al. Mosaicplasty for the treatment of articular defects of the knee and ankle. Clin Orthop 2001;391(Suppl):S328–36.

[12] Ma HL, Hung SC, Wang ST, et al. Osteochondral autografts transfer for post-traumatic osteochondral defect of the knee-2 to 5 years follow-up. Injury 2004;35(12):1286–92.

[13] Nakagawa Y, Matsusue Y, Suzuki T, et al. Osteochondral grafting for cartilage defects in the patellar grooves of bilateral knee joints. Arthroscopy 2004;20(Suppl 2): 32–8.

[14] Ahmad CS, Cohen ZA, Levine WN, et al. Biomechanical and topographic considerations for autologous osteochondral grafting in the knee. Am J Sports Med 2001;29(2):201–6.

[15] Bartz RL, Kamaric E, Noble PC, et al. Topographic matching of selected donor and recipient sites for osteochondral autografting of the articular surface of the femoral condyles. Am J Sports Med 2001;29(2): 207–12.

[16] Terukina M, Fujioka H, Yoshiya S, et al. Analysis of the thickness and curvature of articular cartilage of the femoral condyle. Arthroscopy 2003;19(9): 969–73.

[17] Sanders TG, Mentzer KD, Miller MD, et al. Autogenous osteochondral "plug" transfer for the treatment of focal chondral defects: postoperative MR appearance with clinical correlation. Skeletal Radiol 2001;30(10): 570–8.

[18] Garretson III RB, Katolik LI, Verma N, et al. Contact pressure at osteochondral donor sites in the patellofemoral joint. Am J Sports Med 2004;32(4):967–74.

[19] Duchow J, Hess T, Kohn D. Primary stability of press-fit-implanted osteochondral grafts. Influence of graft size, repeated insertion, and harvesting technique. Am J Sports Med 2000;28(1):24–7.

[20] Diduch DR, Chhabra A, Blessey P, et al. Osteochondral autograft plug transfer: achieving perpendicularity. J Knee Surg 2003;16(1):17–20.

[21] Evans PJ, Miniaci A, Hurtig MB. Manual punch versus power harvesting of osteochondral grafts. Arthroscopy 2004;20(3):306–10.

[22] Kuroki H, Nakagawa Y, Mori K, et al. Mechanical effects of autogenous osteochondral surgical grafting procedures and instrumentation on grafts of articular cartilage. Am J Sports Med 2004;32(3):612–20.

[23] Makino T, Fujioka H, Kurosaka M, et al. Histologic analysis of the implanted cartilage in an exact-fit osteochondral transplantation model. Arthroscopy 2001;17(7):747–51.

[24] Makino T, Fujioka H, Terukina M, et al. The effect of graft sizing on osteochondral transplantation. Arthroscopy 2004;20(8):837–40.

[25] Koh JL, Wirsing K, Lautenschlager E, et al. The effect of graft height mismatch on contact pressure following osteochondral grafting: a biomechanical study. Am J Sports Med 2004;32(2):317–20.

[26] Wu JZ, Herzog W, Hasler EM. Inadequate placement of osteochondral plugs may induce abnormal stress-strain distributions in articular cartilage – finite element simulations. Med Eng Phys 2002;24(2):85–97.

[27] Pearce SG, Hurtig MB, Clarnette R, et al. An investigation of 2 techniques for optimizing joint surface congruency using multiple cylindrical osteochondral autografts. Arthroscopy 2001;17(1):50–5.

[28] Huang FS, Simonian PT, Norman AG, et al. Effects of small incongruities in a sheep model of osteochondral autografting. Am J Sports Med 2004;32(8): 1842–8.

[29] Barber FA, Chow JC. Arthroscopic osteochondral transplantation: histologic results. Arthroscopy 2001; 17(8):832–5.

[30] Lane JG, Massie JB, Ball ST, et al. Follow-up of osteochondral plug transfers in a goat model: a 6-month study. Am J Sports Med 2004;32(6):1440–50.

[31] Simonian PT, Sussmann PS, Wickiewicz TL, et al. Contact pressures at osteochondral donor sites in the knee. Am J Sports Med 1998;26(4):491–4.

[32] Jackson DW, Lalor PA, Aberman HM, et al. Spontaneous repair of full-thickness defects of articular cartilage in a goat model. A preliminary study. J Bone Joint Surg Am 2001;83-A(1):53–64.

[33] Messner K, Gillquist J. Cartilage repair: a critical review. Acta Orthop Scand 1996;67:523–9.

[34] Guettler JH, Demetropoulos CK, Yang KH, et al. Osteochondral defects in the human knee: influence of defect size on cartilage rim stress and load redistribution to surrounding cartilage. Am J Sports Med 2004;32(6):1451–8.

[35] Nakagawa Y, Matsusue Y, Nakamura T. A novel surgical procedure for osteochondritis dissecans of the lateral femoral condyle: exchanging osteochondral plugs taken from donor and recipient sites. Arthroscopy 2002;18(1):E5.

[36] Niederauer GG, Slivka MA, Leatherbury NC, et al. Evaluation of multiphase implants for repair of focal osteochondral defects in goats. Biomaterials 2000; 21:2561–74.

[37] Feczko P, Hangody L, Varga J, et al. Experimental results of donor site filling for autologous osteochondral mosaicplasty. Arthroscopy 2003;19(7):755–61.

[38] Gole MD, Poulsen D, Marzo JM, et al. Chondrocyte viability in press-fit cryopreserved osteochondral allografts. J Orthop Res 2004;22(4):781–7.

[39] Matsusue Y, Kotake T, Nakagawa Y, et al. Arthroscopic osteochondral autograft transplantation for chondral lesion of the tibial plateau of the knee. Arthroscopy 2001;17(6):653–9.

[40] Wang CJ. Treatment of focal articular cartilage lesions of the knee with autogenous osteochondral grafts: a 2- to 4-year follow-up study. Arch Orthop Trauma Surg 2002;122(3):169–72.

[41] Horas U, Pelinkovic D, Herr G, et al. Autologous chondrocyte implantation and osteochondral cylinder transplantation in cartilage repair of the knee joint. A prospective, comparative trial. J Bone Joint Surg Am 2003;85(2):185–92.

ORTHOPEDIC
CLINICS
OF NORTH AMERICA

Orthop Clin N Am 36 (2005) 459–467

Indications for Allografts

Paul E. Caldwell III, MD, Walter R. Shelton, MD*

*Mississippi Sports Medicine and Orthopaedic Center, University of Mississippi of School of Medicine,
1325 East Fortification Street, Jackson, MS 39202, USA*

The use of allografts in orthopaedic knee reconstruction continues to gain popularity. Approximately 1 million musculoskeletal allografts were distributed in the United Sates in 2004 alone. Allografts are used to treat knee ligament instabilities, but have also been used in meniscal and osteochondral transplantation. Allografts have definite advantages, including the lack of donor site morbidity, shorter operative times, ease of sizing, a lack of clinically significant immunologic reactions, and good results in clinical studies [1]. These advantages must be weighed against the potential risks for bacterial and viral infection, which continue to be associated with their use despite modern tissue procurement methods.

History

According to Bolano et al [2], MacEwen first reported the use of allograft bone in 1880. Lexer [3] reported 23 cases of osteoarticular allograft use in the knee between 1908 and 1925. In 1981, Noyes and colleagues [4] and Shino and colleagues [5] reported good results with allograft ligament reconstruction in the knee. In 1989 Milachowski and colleagues [6] reported the first use of human meniscal allografts. These early reports and subsequent studies have

continued to drive the interest and indications for allograft use.

Procurement

In an effort to establish standards and guidelines for the procurement of allografts, the American Association of Tissue Banks (AATB) was founded in 1976. Presently, over 85 tissue banks are AATB accredited worldwide. The AATB first published the "Standards for Tissue Banking" in 1984, which has since undergone numerous revisions. These standards include: (1) obtaining a detailed medical, social, and sexual history [1]; (2) a physical examination with specific attention to hepatosplenomegaly, lymphadenopathy, and the presence of cutaneous lesions [2]; (3) the result of the autopsy (if performed) to be included in the tissue procurement workup [3]; (4) the following tests on donor serum: HIV I and II, hepatitis surface antigen, hepatitis C antibodies, syphilis antibodies, and T-cell lymphotrophic virus antibodies[4]. All of these precautions, along with sterile procurement, facilitate the safety of allograft tissue [7].

A new test, the polymerized chain reaction (PCR), which detects the presence of viral RNA, is more sensitive than antigen/antibody tests. Although not mandated by the AATB or Food and Drug Administration (FDA), PCR testing is being increasingly used because it decreases the window of vulnerability from 4 to 6 weeks to about 10 days. PCR tests for hepatitis C and HIV are available. Surgeons should familiarize themselves with the methods and tests used by their tissue banks before using allografts.

* Corresponding author.
E-mail address: wsheltonMD@msmoc.com
(W.R. Shelton).

0030-5898/05/$ – see front matter © 2005 Elsevier Inc. All rights reserved.
doi:10.1016/j.ocl.2005.05.008

orthopedic.theclinics.com

Sterilization

The potential for viral and bacterial infections continues to be the major disadvantage for allograft use. The Centers for Disease Control and Prevention (CDC) has stated that,

> When possible, a method that can kill bacterial spores should be used to process tissue. Existing sterilization technologies used for tissue allografts, such as gamma irradiation or new technologies effective against bacterial spores, should be considered. Unless a sporicidal method is used, aseptically processed tissue should not be considered sterile, and health-care providers should be informed of the possible risk for bacterial infection [8].

Sterilization techniques that kill virus and bacterial spores completely (eg, heat or high-dose gamma radiation) adversely affect the allograft tissue itself. No perfect method to sterilize grafts while protecting their collagen structure presently exists. A recent death caused by clostridium infection from a contaminated graft has heightened awareness of this problem. The use of low-dose gamma irradiation and antibiotic soaks and washes are secondary sterilization techniques that are effective to varying degrees and do not degrade the biomechanical integrity of the allograft.

Ethylene oxide, when used in a gaseous state, is a successful sterilization method against bacterial and viral particles [9,10]. However, increased graft failure and chronic synovitis are associated with the use of ethylene oxide and have compelled most tissue banks to discontinue its use [11,12].

Gamma irradiation effectively kills bacteria and viruses through direct alteration of nucleic acids and the generation of free radicals [13]. Unfortunately, gamma irradiation alters the biomechanical integrity of allograft tissue at doses high enough to kill bacteria and viruses [14]. Currently, 2.5 mrad is the recommended maximum dose to provide maximal bacterial eradication without significantly altering the biomechanical structure of the allograft. Because higher doses are required to kill spores and viruses, the effectiveness of this technique is limited [15,16]. Techniques such as antibiotic soaking are limited by tissue infiltration. The FDA has validated innovative low-temperature chemical sterilization techniques that are effective against spores and viruses, and which hold the promise for the future [17,18]. The most common method of ensuring sterile grafts is through sterile harvest and processing with low-dose gamma irradiation to kill surface pathogens. Surgeons should familiarize themselves with the processes used by the tissue banks that provide their allografts.

Storage

Allografts are stored by one of the following methods: fresh allograft, fresh freezing, cryopreservation, or freeze drying. Fresh allografts must be implanted 24 to 48 hours after harvest, whereas freezing fresh allografts at -80°C to -196°C allows storage for up to 3 to 5 years—a process that kills donor cells. Cryopreservation controls the rate of freezing while the water is chemically extracted, allowing up to 80% of the cells to remain viable. Freeze drying or lyophilization involves removing up to 95% of the moisture and subsequent vacuum packaging. This process allows storage at room temperature for up to 3 to 5 years and requires rehydration before implantation [19].

Risk for disease transmission

Despite all of the precautions taken during the process of allograft tissue preparation, the risk for disease transmission remains a concern to surgeon and patient. Clostridium spores are not killed by present sterilization measures and have been implicated in at least 13 cases of infection—one fatal in 2001 [8]. Infections have been reported after the use of ligament, meniscal, and articular cartilage allografts.

Three cases of HIV transmission through allograft have been reported since the inception of universal donor testing in 1985 [20]. The risk for acquiring HIV after proper screening and testing has been estimated to be approximately 1 in 1.6 million [21]. Hepatitis C virus (HCV) has also been reported with allograft use. In a recent report of 38 patients receiving allograft tissue from one infected donor, at least six patients actually tested positive for HCV [22]. In 2002, The American Academy of Orthopaedic Surgeons formed the Tissue Banking Project Team (TBPT) in response to these recent reports. The objective of the TBPT is to work in association with the FDA and CDC to make the practice of allograft tissue preparation and distribution a more uniform and safer process [23]. Even though steps have been taken to enhance the safety of allografts, risks for disease transmission continue to be present and patients should be educated during the consent process.

Physiology of incorporation

The incorporation of the allograft into the host is the final step for achieving a viable and functioning structure. Once implanted, allografts are a scaffold for host tissue ingrowth [19]. Allografts progress through four stages of healing: cell necrosis, revascularization, cellular repopulation, and remodeling. Cell death occurs from the time of harvest, through procurement, and shortly after implantation. Revascularization occurs with the ingrowth of host blood vessels and is closely followed by cellular repopulation. These initial three stages occur swiftly, and have been shown to be complete in as early as 4 weeks in the goat model [24]. Remodeling, which includes fibroblast proliferation and collagen synthesis, may take up to 18 months to complete, and is primarily responsible for the biointegrity of the graft. Jackson and colleagues [25] have demonstrated that allograft tissue remodels slower and takes longer to regain strength than autograft tissue. Fromm and colleagues [26,27] have shown that deep frozen and cryopreserved allograft tendons will reinnervate by 24 weeks in the rabbit model. Functionally, several studies have compared ACL allografts and autografts and found no clinical differences [1,28,29].

Ligament allografts

History

A stable knee is necessary for optimal function and preservation of menisci and articular cartilage [30]. Anterior cruciate ligament (ACL) tears are the most common functional knee instability. Approximately 100,000 ACL reconstructions are performed annually in the United States. Most patients who desire to return to cutting and pivoting activities require reconstruction. The search for an ideal graft continues and has included zenografts and synthetics. Autografts and allografts remain the most commonly selected because of the consistently good results achieved.

Indications

Surgeons and patients should consider all the pros and cons when choosing a graft. The patient's age and activity level together with the availability of a quality autograft and the surgeon's preference and experience should be considerations. Although autograft bone-patellar-tendon-bone (BPTB) is still the most common graft used for ACL reconstruction, anterior knee pain, patellar fracture, patellar tendon rupture, and quadriceps weakness have been reported. Hamstring and quadriceps tendon grafts also have graft site morbidity. The absence of donor site morbidity is the major advantage of using an allograft. This advantage should be weighed against the risk for disease transmission, increased cost, and increased time of graft incorporation. Older patients, low activity level, revision or multiligament surgery, skeletal immaturity, patellofemoral pain, kneeling occupation or sport, patient preference, and surgeon experience are all indications for allograft selection [31,32]. Other ligaments, including the posterior cruciate, medial collateral ligament, lateral collateral ligament, and patellar tendon, have been reconstructed successfully with allografts.

Surgical considerations

Surgical techniques and principals are similar for allografts and autografts. One difference between the two is the remodeling phase of allograft incorporation. Cordrey and colleagues [33] have established in the animal model that allografts take longer to remodel. Animal studies have demonstrated that after 1 year the vascular and fibrous histologic patterns in BPTB allografts are similar to those of the native ligament [25,34–36]. Shino and colleagues [5] have demonstrated with second-look arthroscopy that human allografts reach histologic maturity within the first 18 months and remain unchanged as viable ligaments thereafter. Although the gross and histologic appearance of allografts appear to be similar to the native ACL, the strength of the allograft has been reported to be 27% to 90% of that of the native ACL in the animal model [25,36,37]. Despite the lack of conclusive evidence regarding the tensile strength of allograft tissue during remodeling, clinical studies have failed to demonstrate an increased rate of failure [38]. Because of this uncertainty, some surgeons elect to protect allograft reconstructions longer during the postoperative rehabilitation [31].

Clinical results

Most clinical studies using allografts have been with BPTB reconstruction of the ACL. Harner and colleagues [1] found no difference in patient symptoms, stability, activity level, and functional outcomes between allograft and autograft ACL BPTB reconstructions at 3- to 5-year follow-up. These findings were substantiated by Shelton and colleagues [28], who compared allograft and autograft ACL BPTB reconstruction with a minimum follow-up of 24 months and found no difference regarding pain, effusion, stability, range of motion, patellofemoral crepitus, and thigh circumference. Westerheide and colleagues [29] compared outcomes of patients receiving autograft patellar tendon and allograft patellar tendon at

8 to 14 years and found no significant differences in subjective or objective parameters. The results of the study by Indelli and colleagues [39] with cryopreserved Achilles tendon allograft in primary ACL reconstruction in 50 athletes with 3- to 5-year follow-up found 92% returned to their previous level of sport. Reconstruction of the posterior cruciate ligament using an Achilles allograft has been reported by Fanelli and Edson [40]. Their results show excellent restoration of stability and emphasize the advantages of an allograft when large strong grafts are needed.

Summary

Although the ideal graft for ligament reconstruction does not exist at this time, allografts are an accepted alternative to autograft. When selecting a graft, the advantages and disadvantages of allografts should be considered. During the consent process, comprehensive patient education is imperative to assist in the decision-making process.

Articular cartilage allografts

History

Mechanical loading is essential for the homeostasis of articular cartilage. When this threshold is exceeded, injury may occur and the capacity to heal is limited by the avascular environment. Chondral lesions generate an irregular surface that predisposes the joint to meniscal tears and early degenerative arthritis. Not all chondral lesions are symptomatic, requiring operative intervention [41]. When operative intervention is indicated, several options exist, including lavage and debridement, and bone marrow stimulation. These procedures are less than ideal, resulting in the production of a biomechanically inferior fibrocartilage consisting of predominately type I collagen. Osteochondral autografts, transplantation of autologous cartilage cells, and osteochondral allografts are optional methods used to fill isolated articular defects [42].

Indications

Factors that must be assessed when deciding on the treatment of a full thickness focal cartilage defect include location, size, and depth of the defect; age and activity of the patient; the condition of the surrounding articular cartilage; meniscal integrity; ligament instability; limb alignment; and a history of inflammatory arthropathies [43]. The risk associated

with allografts must be weighed against the lack of donor-site morbidity and size restrictions placed on autografts when planning treatment. Another advantage of an articular allograft is the ability to harvest from a younger donor who has healthier cartilage than the recipient. The ideal patient to treat with an osteochondral allograft is similar to that of an autograft, with the exception of the defect size. Most surgeons restrict the use of autografts to lesions under 2 cm because of the limited availability of donor autograft sites and the potential for donor-site morbidity [31]. Treating isolated defects, such as osteochondritis dissecans or traumatic defects, is important to the success of osteochondral allograft transplantation. Rheumatoid arthritis, generalized osteoarthritis involving both sides of the joint, and corticosteroid-induced osteonecrosis should all be considered relative contraindications for an osteochondral allograft [44]. Most reported cases involve allograft transplantation for lesions of the femur, but the tibia, patella, and other joints have also been successfully treated.

Surgical considerations

Because most osteochondral allografts are implanted as fresh grafts to preserve chondrocyte viability, the risks for disease transmission and immunologic reaction are greater. The shorter time between harvest and implantation also makes sizing more difficult [45,46]. Czitrom and colleagues [47] have demonstrated that human chondrocytes are viable and metabolically active at 12 and 72 months after implantation in fresh grafts. Pearsall and colleagues [48] and Williams and colleagues [49] have recently shown that refrigerated osteochondral allografts can be preserved for up to 45 days with over half of the chondrocyte viability maintained. To avoid these problems, cryopreserved articular grafts have been used because they have greater storage time, are less immunogenic, and preserve up to 80% viability of cells. One should try to implant an osteochondral allograft with the highest population of viable chondrocytes, while placing the patient at the least possible risk.

Sizing osteochondral allografts has also been a technical problem. Commonly, grafts are dowel or shell grafts, depending on the size of the lesion. Dowel grafts are easily prepared, inserted by press-fit, and are applicable for lesions up to 35 mm in diameter. These cylindrical grafts are commonly used for well-circumscribed lesions of the femur and patella. Shell grafts, on the other hand, are not limited by the size or shape of the lesion, typically are templated and hand crafted to match the size and contour of the defect, and require supplemental fixation. They are more commonly employed for lesions in the posterior femur or tibial plateau. With both techniques, the normal contour of the joint must be recreated to ensure optimal incorporation and function [50].

Patients are placed on restricted weight-bearing and early motion is encouraged during the initial postoperative period. The duration of restricted weight-bearing depends on the type and location of the graft, and radiographic evidence of healing. Most patients return to unrestricted activity by 6 months with femoral grafts and 1 year with tibial plateau grafts [51].

Clinical results

Most results of osteochondral allografts have been documented using fresh osteochondral allografts. Ghazavi and colleagues [52] reported on 108 of 126 knees that had a good or excellent result for femoral defects secondary to trauma or osteochondral defect (OCD) at an average follow-up of 7.5 years. They documented an allograft survival of 95% at 5 years, 71% at 10 years, and 66% at 20 years. Bugbee and Convery [53] reported on 97 patients who were evaluated based on the number of surfaces grafted. The mean follow-up was 50 months and the results were good or excellent for 86% of the single surfaces grafted and 53% for two opposing articulating surfaces grafted. They concluded that results depend on the number and area of surfaces replaced and that inferior outcomes are associated with a poor allograft fit, large defects, and replacing more than one chondral surface. Garrett [54] reviewed 17 patients at an average of 3.5 years who were treated with a fresh osteochondral allograft for osteochondritis desiccans lesions of the lateral femoral condyle. They reported that 16 of the 17 patients were asymptomatic, and that radiographs confirmed bony incorporation of the graft. Cryopreserved osteochondral allografts yield inferior results compared with fresh allografts [55,56].

Summary

Because articular cartilage has a limited ability to heal, multiple options for treatment of chondral lesions have emerged. Despite the concerns of disease transmission, expense, limited availability, and immunogenic reactions, osteochondral allografts play an important role in the treatment of defects measuring more than 2.5 cm. Fresh allografts have the best results, whereas cryopreserved grafts maintain a viable population of cells and minimize risks associated with allografts. Advances in gene therapy and tissue engineering may generate the ideal graft source for cartilage lesions in the future.

Meniscal allografts

History

Treatment of meniscal injury has evolved from total meniscectomy toward meniscal preservation and repair. In 1948, the article by Fairbank [57] showed detrimental radiographic consequences of total meniscectomy. The meniscus is fundamental to preserving normal articular cartilage in the knee [58–60]. Not all meniscal injuries are repairable, and total meniscectomy may be required. The natural history of arthritis in the meniscus-deficient knee has led to the development of allograft meniscal transplantation.

Arnoczky and colleagues [61] established the possibility of meniscal allograft transplantation in the dog model and Milachowski and colleagues [6] reported the first clinical results in 1989. Interest in meniscal allograft transplantation has increased since then.

Indications

Indications for allograft meniscal transplant continue to evolve. The ideal candidate is physiologically young and has a history of a total meniscectomy and subsequent pain localized to the appropriate tibiofemoral compartment. Limb malalignment and ligamentous instability must be addressed before, or concurrent with, the transplantation. Radiographs, MRI, and arthroscopy may be needed to ensure that the articular surfaces are without significant wear. Many authors recommend grade II Outerbridge changes or better, but controversy remains regarding focal lesions [31,62]. The patient should also be assessed for compliance and realistic expectations to ensure the potential success of the operation. Absolute contraindications include obesity; rheumatoid arthritis; metabolic diseases such as gout; and infectious disease. Prophylactic meniscal allograft transplantation to prevent potential degenerative changes in asymptomatic young active patients who have undergone a total meniscectomy has been recommended, but remains controversial [63].

Surgical considerations

Proper meniscal sizing is essential for successful transplantation and is most commonly accomplished by plain radiograph with a reference marker. MRI and CT may also be used to ensure correct sizing [64–67].

Fresh-frozen or cryopreserved grafts are the most popular choices for allograft meniscal transplantation. Cryopreservation does allow extended storage while preserving viable cells and the integrity of the basement membrane, but is an expensive process. Rapid repopulation of the graft by host cells has led to the use of fresh-frozen grafts [68]. Freezing of fresh tissue is less expensive and diminishes the potential for an immune response.

Arthroscopic-assisted allograft meniscal transplantation has lowered cost and surgical morbidity, but requires advanced arthroscopic skills [69]. Proper bony fixation of the meniscal horns is required to prevent peripheral extrusion of the meniscus during weight-bearing. Bylski-Austrow and colleagues [70] have supported this concept by analyzing the biomechanical properties of the graft in the animal model. Implantation is commonly accomplished by means of bone plugs or the "keyhole technique." Peripheral healing and revascularization are accomplished by adequate debridement of any meniscal remnant to a bleeding rim, and by secure peripheral suturing. Rehabilitation consists of full range of motion immediately after surgery and limited weight-bearing for 6 weeks [71].

Clinical results

In 1989, Milachowski and colleagues [6] first published their experience with fresh-frozen and freeze-dried grafts in 22 patients at an average of 14 months. They performed second-look arthroscopy to establish peripheral healing in 15 of 18 grafts. Garrett [62] later reported on 43 patients who had a 2- to 7-year follow-up. Most of their patients underwent additional procedures at the time of transplantation, and only six had an isolated meniscal transplant. Of these patients, 15 were asymptomatic and had a good clinical outcome. Twenty-eight second-look arthroscopies were performed, with 20 showing good healing and eight failures credited to grade IV articular changes.

In 1995 Noyes and Barber-Westin [72] reported on a group of 96 fresh-frozen irradiated grafts in 82 patients. Their failure rate was greater than 50% because of the high rate of grade IV arthrosis and failure to anchor both horns of the menisci with bony attachments. Of these grafts, 29 had to be removed before 2 years. Stollsteimer and colleagues [71] followed 22 patients (23 knees) who had nonirradiated, cryopreserved allografts for an average of 40 months and found improved International Knee Documentation Committee (IKDC), Lysholm, and Tegner scores. The most significant improvement was found to be in pain relief following transplant. Meniscal shrinkage was a concern following MRI evaluation of 12 patients at 24 months. Wirth and colleagues [73] reported long-term results of up to 14 years on 23 patients who underwent meniscal allograft transplantation combined with ACL reconstruction. Patients were evaluated clinically with Lysholm scores, radiographs, MRI, arthrography, and arthroscopy. The six patients who had deep-frozen transplants had better results than the 17 who had lyophilized transplants. Noyes and colleagues [74] recently evaluated 40 cryopreserved meniscal allografts in 38 symptomatic patients under the age of 50. Most of these patients underwent supplementary procedures, including osteochondral autograft transfer and ligament reconstruction. They were evaluated at a mean of 40 months and 89% rated their knees improved. Although good to excellent clinical results have been demonstrated in a diverse group of patients, additional studies are needed to establish the long-term functionality of meniscal allografts and their role in preventing potential cartilage degeneration.

Summary

The role of allograft meniscal transplantation in the treatment of the postmeniscectomized knee has yet to be completely defined. The indications for transplantation continue to evolve and will be established by future controlled studies. The advent of arthroscopic-assisted transplantation has lowered the cost and surgical morbidity, but the risks associated with allograft transplantation remain. In the future, research may provide methods of meniscal regeneration, but transplantation remains the current standard.

Summary

Technology has made the use of allograft tissue transplantation a common procedure in today's orthopaedic practice. Although the use of allografts continues to increase and screening tests have reduced the risks, certain precautions should be followed. A comprehensive discussion with the patient and family members is imperative. The risks, benefits, and alternatives must be clearly explained during the consent process. The surgeon must be familiar with the tissue provider's banking process and the origin of the particular graft. Excellent results have been demonstrated using allograft ligament, osteochondral, and meniscal tissue, but the goal remains to provide the patient with the best graft choice accompanied by the least amount of risk.

References

[1] Harner CD, Olson E, Irrgang JJ, et al. Allograft versus autograft anterior cruciate ligament reconstruction: 3- to 5-year outcome. Clin Orthop 1996;324:134–44.

[2] Bolano L, Kopta JA. The immunology of bone and cartilage transplantation. Orthopedics 1991;14:987–96.

[3] Lexer E. Joint transplantations and arthroplasty. Surg Gynecol Obstet 1925;40:782–809.

[4] Noyes FR, Barber SD, Mangine RE. Bone-patellar ligament-bone and fascia lata allografts for reconstruction of the anterior cruciate ligament. J Bone Joint Surg Am 1990;72:1125–36.

[5] Shino K, Inoue M, Horibe S, et al. Maturation of allograft tendons transplanted into the knee: an arthroscopic and histological study. J Bone Joint Surg Br 1988;70:556–60.

[6] Milachowski KA, Weismeier K, Wirth CJ. Homologous meniscus transplantation: experimental and clinical results. Int Orthop 1989;13:1–11.

[7] Hornicek FJ, Woll JE, Kasprisin D. Standards for tissue banking. 10th edition. McLean (VA): American Association of Tissue Banks; 2002.

[8] Centers for Disease Control and Prevention. Update: allograft associated bacterial infections—United States, 2002. MMWR Morb Mortal Wkly Rep 2002; 51:207–10.

[9] Phillips CR, Kaye S. The sterilizing action of gaseous ethylene oxide: I. Review. Am J Hyg 1949;50:270–9.

[10] Jordy A, Hoff-Jorgensen R, Flagstad A, et al. Virus inactivation by ethylene oxide containing gases. Acta Vet Scand 1975;16:379–87.

[11] Jackson DW, Windler GE, Simon TM. Intraarticular reaction associated with the use of freeze-dried, ethylene oxide-sterilized bone-patella tendon-bone allografts in the reconstruction of the anterior cruciate ligament. Am J Sports Med 1990;18:1–10.

[12] Roberts TS, Drez Jr D, McCarthy W, et al. Anterior cruciate ligament reconstruction using freeze-dried, ethylene oxide-sterilized, bone-patellar tendon-bone allografts. Two year results in thirty-six patients. Am J Sports Med 1991;19:35–41.

[13] Hansen JM, Shaffer HL. Sterilization and preservation by radiation sterilization. In: Block SS, editor. Disinfection, sterilization, and preservation. 5th edition. Philadelphia: Lippincott, Williams & Wilkins; 2001. p. 729–46.

[14] Bright R, Smars J, Gambill V. Sterilization of human bone by irradiation. In: Friedlaender GE, Mankin HJ, Sell KW, editors. Osteochondral allografts: biology, banking, and clinical applications. National Institute of Allergy and Infectious Diseases (US) & AAOT Banks. Boston: Little Brown; 1983. p. 223–32.

[15] Fideler BM, Vangsness Jr CT, Moore T, et al. Effects of gamma irradiation on the human immunodeficiency virus. A study in frozen human bone-patellar ligament-bone grafts obtained from infected cadavera. J Bone Joint Surg Am 1994;76:1032–5.

[16] Campbell DG, Li P. Sterilization of HIV with irradiation: relevance to infected bone allografts. Aust N Z J Surg 1999;69:517–21.

[17] Regeneration Technologies. The biocleanse tissue sterilization process: a proven standard for tissue safety. Gainesville (FL): Regeneration Technologies; 2003.

[18] Summitt M, Bianchi J, Keesling J, et al. Bomechanical testing of bone treated through a new tissue cleaning process. In: 25th Annual Meeting of the American Association of Tissue Banks. Washington (DC): American Association of Tissue Banks; 2001. p. 55, s-15.

[19] Shelton WR, Treacy SH, Dukes AD, et al. Use of allografts in knee reconstruction: I. Basic science aspects and current status. J Am Acad Orthop Surg 1998; 6:165–8.

[20] Simonds RJ, Holmberg SD, Hurwitz RL, et al. Transmission of human immunodeficiency virus type 1 from a seronegative organ and tissue donor. N Engl J Med 1992;326:726–32.

[21] Buck BE, Malinin TI, Brown MD. Bone transplantation and human immunodeficiency virus: an estimate of risk of acquired immunodeficiency syndrome (AIDS). Clin Orthop 1989;240:129–36.

[22] Tugwell BD, Williams IT, Thomas AR, et al. Hepatitis C virus (HCV) transmission to tissue and organ recipients from an antibody-negative donor. Presented at the Interscience Conference on Antimicrobial Agents and Chemotherapy. San Diego, September 27–30, 2002.

[23] Kennedy J. American Academy of Orthopaedic Surgeons Bulletin April 2003 Volume 51, No.2: AAOS acts on tissue banking recommendations, Allograft tissue safety. Available at: http://www.aaos.org/wordhtml/bulletin/apr03/acdnws8.htm. Accessed December 1, 2004.

[24] Jackson DW, Simon TM, Kurzweil PR, et al. Survival of cells after intraarticular transplantation of fresh allografts of the patellar and anterior cruciate ligaments: DNA-probe analysis in a goat model. J Bone Joint Surg Am 1992;74:112–8.

[25] Jackson DW, Grood ES, Arnoczky SP, et al. Freeze dried anterior cruciate ligament allografts: preliminary studies in a goat model. Am J Sports Med 1987;15: 295–303.

[26] Fromm B, Schafer B, Kummer W. Nerve supply to the anterior cruciate ligament and cruciate ligament allograft. Sportverletz Sportschaden 1993;7(3):101–8.

[27] Fromm B, Schafer B, Parsch D, et al. Reconstruction

of the anterior cruciate ligament with a cryopreserved ACL allograft. A microangiographic and immunohistochemical study in rabbits. Int Orthop 1996;20(6): 378–82.

[28] Shelton WR, Papendick L, Dukes AD. Autograft versus allograft anterior cruciate ligament reconstruction. Arthroscopy 1997;13:446–9.

[29] Westerheide KJ, Fluhme DJ, Francis KA, et al. Long term follow up of allograft versus autograft bone patellar tendon bone ACL reconstruction. Presented at the American Orthopaedic Society for Sports Medicine. Orlando, 2002.

[30] Rovere GD, Adair DM. Anterior cruciate-deficient knees: a review of the literature. Am J Sports Med 1983;11(6):412–9.

[31] Rihn JA, Harner CD. The use of musculoskeletal allograft tissue in knee surgery. Arthroscopy 2003; 19(Suppl 1):51–66.

[32] Strickland SM, MacGillivray JD, Warren RF. Anterior cruciate ligament reconstruction with allograft tendons. Orthop Clin North Am 2003;34(1):41–7.

[33] Cordrey LJ, McCorkle H, Hilton E. A comparative study of fresh autogenous and preserved homogenous tendon grafts in rabbits. J Bone Joint Surg Br 1963;45: 182–95.

[34] Shino K, Kawasaki T, Hirose H, et al. Replacement of the anterior cruciate ligament by an allogeneic tendon graft: an experimental study in the dog. J Bone Joint Surg Br 1984;66:672–81.

[35] Arnoczky SP, Warren RF, Ashlock MA. Replacement of the anterior cruciate ligament using a patellar tendon allograft: an experimental study. J Bone Joint Surg Am 1986;68:376–85.

[36] Drez Jr DJ, DeLee J, Holden JP, et al. Anterior cruciate ligament reconstruction using bone-patellar tendon-bone allografts: a biological and biomechanical evaluation in goats. Am J Sports Med 1991;19:256–63.

[37] Nikolaou PK, Seaber AV, Glisson RR, et al. Anterior cruciate ligament allograft transplantation: Long-term function, histology, revascularization, and operative technique. Am J Sports Med 1986;14:348–60.

[38] Noyes FR, Barber SD. The effect of an extra-articular procedure on allograft reconstructions for chronic ruptures of the anterior cruciate ligament. J Bone Joint Surg Am 1991;73:882–92.

[39] Indelli PF, Dillingham MF, Fanton GS, et al. Anterior cruciate ligament reconstruction using cryopreserved allografts. Clin Orthop 2004;Mar(420):268–75.

[40] Fanelli GC, Edson CJ. Combined posterior cruciate ligament-posterolateral reconstructions with Achilles tendon allograft and biceps femoris tendon tenodesis: 2- to 10-year follow-up. Arthroscopy 2004;20(4): 339–45.

[41] Curl WW, Krome J, Gordon ES, et al. Cartilage injuries: a review of 31,516 knee arthroscopies. Arthroscopy 1997;13:456–60.

[42] Jackson DW, Scheer MJ, Simon TM. Cartilage substitutes: overview of basic science and treatment options. J Am Acad Orthop Surg 2001;9:37–52.

[43] Sgaglione N, Miniaci A, Gillogly S, et al. Update on advanced surgical techniques in the treatment of traumatic focal articular cartilage lesions in the knee. Arthroscopy 2002;18:9–32.

[44] Shelton WR, Treacy SH, Dukes AD, et al. Use of allografts in knee reconstruction: II. Surgical considerations. J Am Acad Orthop Surg 1998;6(3):169–75.

[45] Stevenson S, Shaffer JW, Goldberg VM. The humoral response to vascular and nonvascular allografts of bone. Clin Orthop 1996;323:56–95.

[46] Strong DM, Friedlaender GE, Tomford WW, et al. Immunologic responses in human recipients of osseous osteochondral allografts. Clin Orthop 1996;326: 107–14.

[47] Czitrom AA, Keating S, Gross AE. The viability of articular cartilage in fresh osteochondral allografts after clinical transplantation. J Bone Joint Surg Am 1990; 72:574–81.

[48] Pearsall IV AW, Tucker JA, Hester RB, et al. Chondrocyte viability in refrigerated osteochondral allografts used for transplantation within the knee. Am J Sports Med 2004;32(1):125–31.

[49] Williams III RJ, Dreese JC, Chen CT. Chondrocyte survival and material properties of hypothermically stored cartilage: an evaluation of tissue used for osteochondral allograft transplantation. Am J Sports Med 2004;32(1):132–9.

[50] Pearce SG, Hurtig MB, Clarnette R, et al. An investigation of 2 techniques for optimizing joint surface congruency using multiple cylindrical osteochondral autografts. Arthroscopy 2001;17:50–5.

[51] McGuire DA, Carter TR, Shelton WR. Complex knee reconstruction: osteotomies, ligament reconstruction, transplants, and cartilage treatment options. Arthroscopy 2002;18(9 Suppl 2):90–103.

[52] Ghazavi MT, Pritzker KP, Davis AM, et al. Fresh osteochondral allografts for post-traumatic osteochondral defects of the knee. J Bone Joint Surg Br 1997;79: 1008–13.

[53] Bugbee WD, Convery FR. Osteochondral allograft transplantation. Clin Sports Med 1999;18(1):67–75.

[54] Garrett JC. Fresh osteochondral allografts for treatment of articular defects in osteochondritis dissecans of the lateral femoral condyle in adults. Clin Orthop 1994; 303:33–7.

[55] Flynn JM, Springfield DS, Mankin HJ. Osteoarticular allografts to treat distal femoral osteonecrosis. Clin Orthop 1994;303:38–43.

[56] Bakay A, Csonge L, Papp G, et al. Osteochondral resurfacing of the knee joint with allograft: clinical analysis of 33 cases. Int Orthop 1998;22:277–81.

[57] Fairbank TJ. Knee joint changes after meniscectomy. J Bone Joint Surg Br 1948;30:664–70.

[58] Levy IM, Torzilli PA, Gould JD, et al. The effect of lateral meniscectomy on motion of the knee. J Bone Joint Surg Am 1989;71:401–6.

[59] Aagaard H, Verdonk R. Function of the normal meniscus and consequences of meniscal resection. Scand J Med Sci Sports 1999;9:134–40.

[60] Allen CR, Wong EK, Livesay GA, et al. Importance of the medial meniscus in the anterior cruciate ligament-deficient knee. J Orthop Res 2000;18:109–15.

[61] Arnoczky SP, McDevitt CA, Schmidt MB, et al. The effect of cryopreservation on canine menisci: a biochemical, morphologic, and biomechanical evaluation. J Orthop Res 1988;6:1–12.

[62] Garrett JC. Meniscal transplantation: a review of 43 cases with 2- to 7-year follow up. Sports Med Arthrosc Rev 1993;1:164–7.

[63] Johnson DL, Bealle D. Meniscal allograft transplantation. Clin Sports Med 1999;18:93–108.

[64] Garrett JC, Stevensen RN. Meniscal transplantation in the human knee. A preliminary report. Arthroscopy 1991;7:57–62.

[65] Carpenter JE, Wojitys EM, Huston LJ. Preoperative sizing of meniscal allografts. Arthroscopy 1993;9:344.

[66] Pollard ME, Kang Q, Berg EE. Radiographic sizing for meniscal transplantation. Arthroscopy 1995;11:684–7.

[67] Shaffer B, Kennedy S, Klimkiewicz J, et al. Preoperative sizing of meniscal allografts in meniscus transplantation. Am J Sports Med 2000;28:524–33.

[68] Jackson DW, Whelan J, Simon TM. Cell survival after transplantation of fresh meniscal allografts: DNA probe analysis in a goat model. Am J Sports Med 1993;21:540–50.

[69] Shelton WR, Dukes AD. Meniscus replacement with bone anchors: a surgical technique. Arthroscopy 1994;10:324–7.

[70] Bylski-Austrow DI, Meade T, Malumed J. Irradiated meniscal allografts: mechanical and histological studies in the goat. Trans Orthop Res Soc 1992;17:175.

[71] Stollsteimer GT, Shelton WR, Dukes A, et al. Meniscal allograft transplantation: a 1-to 5-year follow-up of 22 patients. Arthroscopy 2000;16:343–7.

[72] Noyes FR, Barber-Westin SD. Irradiated meniscal allografts in the human knee: a two to five year followup. Orthop Trans 1995;19:417.

[73] Wirth CJ, Peters G, Milachowski KA, et al. Long-term results of meniscal allograft transplantation. Am J Sports Med 2002;30(2):174–81.

[74] Noyes FR, Barber-Westin SD, Rankin M. Meniscal transplantation in symptomatic patients less than fifty years old. J Bone Joint Surg Am 2004;86(7):1392–404.

ELSEVIER
SAUNDERS

Orthop Clin N Am 36 (2005) 469 – 484

ORTHOPEDIC
CLINICS
OF NORTH AMERICA

The Indications and Technique for Meniscal Transplant

Winslow Alford, MD[a], Brian J. Cole, MD, MBA[b],*

[a]West Bay Orthopedics, 120 Centerville Road, Warwick, RI 02886-6919, USA
[b]Rush University, Section of Sports Medicine, 1725 West Harrison, Suite 1063, Chicago, IL 60612, USA

Meniscal allograft transplantation (MAT) has moved into mainstream orthopedics. With proper patient selection, and recognition and treatment of comorbid conditions, MAT offers a solution that can at least temporarily decrease pain and increase function. This article reviews the basic science of meniscal mechanics, the pathomechanics of meniscal injury, and MAT indications and techniques. A brief description of treatment of comorbid conditions and the outcomes of MAT is also provided.

Meniscal anatomy and biomechanics

In a healthy knee, the medial and lateral menisci contribute to the health and mechanical protection of articular cartilage and help prevent degenerative joint disease. Removal of or injury to menisci has been implicated in articular degeneration and the development of osteoarthritis [1]. Articular cartilage damage has been shown to occur as early as 12 weeks after meniscectomy in skeletally mature mongrel dogs [2]. The many functions of the menisci include shock absorption, load transmission, secondary mechanical stability, and joint lubrication and nutrition [3].

Menisci are semilunar, wedge-shaped structures that enhance tibial-femoral joint stability by filling the void created by the incongruous femoral condyles and tibial plateau [4]. The lateral meniscus forms a C-shaped incomplete semicircle, whereas the medial meniscus is more U shaped with a wider separation of its anterior and posterior horns than in the lateral

meniscus. By deepening the tibial socket, menisci act as secondary stabilizers—particularly the posterior horn of the medial meniscus, which blocks anterior translation of the tibia on the femur [5–8]. Loss of the posterior horn of the medial meniscus in the setting of primary anterior cruciate ligament (ACL) reconstruction has been associated with graft elongation and joint laxity [9,10], which may ultimately accelerate osteoarthritis in the ACL-deficient knee [5,11].

During the normal gait pattern, the articular surface of the knee bears up to six times the body weight, with over 70% of that load borne by the medial tibial plateau [12,13]. The menisci increase the contact area and dissipate the compressive forces at the articular cartilage. The lateral meniscus carries 70% of the lateral compartment load, compared with just 40% by the medial meniscus [14]. By converting joint-loading forces to radial-directed hoop stresses on circumferential collagen fibers, the menisci transmit 50% of the joint load when the knee is in extension, and 90% when the knee is in flexion [15,16]. Meniscal loss increases peak articular contact stresses and can lead to the development of early degenerative changes [15,17,18]. Loss of just 20% of a meniscus can lead to a 350% increase in contact forces [19]. MAT with bone anchorage of the anterior and posterior horns improves contact forces compared with total meniscectomy [18,21,29] and can protect articular cartilage [22,23].

Meniscus ultrastructure

Meniscal tissue is composed of elongated cells on the surface and ovoid cells in deeper layers that are equipped with few mitochondria, suggesting anaero-

---

* Corresponding author.
E-mail address: bcole@rushortho.com (B.J. Cole).

0030-5898/05/$ – see front matter © 2005 Elsevier Inc. All rights reserved.
doi:10.1016/j.ocl.2005.05.003

orthopedic.theclinics.com

bic metabolism [19]. The extracellular matrix of menisci is 74% water by weight, but type I collagen comprises about 65% of the dry weight, and glycosaminoglycans make up 2% of the dry weight. Other collagens (types II, III, V, and VI) make up about 5% of the dry weight. Elastin, fibronectin, and thromboplastin assist in organizing the matrix by binding molecules. This blood supply of a meniscus is key to successful meniscal repair or transplantation. The inferior medial and lateral geniculate arteries form a plexus encompassing 10% to 30% of the width of the medial meniscus and 10% to 25% of the width of the lateral meniscus [24], combined with a 1- to 3-mm cuff of vascular synovium. Synovial fluid is pumped through a network of micropores during normal joint motion, providing nutrition to articular cartilage [25].

Meniscal tissue is structured as a fiber-reinforced, porous-permeable composite material containing solid (matrix proteins) and fluid (water) [26,27]. Circumferential peripheral collagen bundles act as structural scaffolding of the meniscus, provide hoop stress resistance to strain, and provide increased stiffness. In contrast, the central two thirds has randomly oriented collagen fibers and a sheetlike arrangement of radial tie fibers, with correspondingly higher strain rates and less stiffness [28]. The restraining collagen fibers, if undamaged, permit little swelling in the stiff peripheral region. The less-stiff central region has a high proteoglycan/collagen ratio that promotes hydration and swelling, enabling the meniscus cartilage to load-share with the articular cartilage. Abnormal meniscal hydration pressure indicates collagen or proteoglycan damage.

Collagen and proteoglycan damage can be caused by mechanical factors (tears or surgical resection), enzymatic degradation, or synthesis of new, poorly functioning molecules. Collagen damage leads to abnormal hydration and an irreversible cascade of tissue alteration. When proteoglycans are damaged (but the collagen remains intact), these tissue changes are reversible. For example, immobilization leads to proteoglycan loss, which is reversed after a return of motion stimulates fibrochondrocytes to synthesize new proteoglycan molecules. Central and peripheral tears occur with different mechanisms and have different consequences. With its higher strain rate and lack of stiffness, central meniscus collagen meshwork tears are common (bucket handle tears), often with low-energy mechanisms. Reparability depends on the location and orientation of the tear. The consequence of central tissue resection is far less than that of peripheral meniscal resection. Hoop-strain resistance to joint compression of the meniscus relies on an intact periphery, and tears that violate the peripheral rim can render that compartment meniscus deficient, wherein meniscal allograft transplantation (MAT) may be indicated [29].

These principles also apply to a transplanted meniscus. If a meniscus is transplanted into a degenerative compartment with Fairbank changes [30] or an inflammatory [31] environment, then the allograft will fail as did the native meniscus. Circumferential collagen bundles in the allograft must be intact from anterior to posterior horn with secure bone fixation [18,21,32], using either bone plugs or a slot and keyhole technique. Physiologic loads will stimulate the fibrochondrocytes. Proper load-sharing and congruent articulation require correct allograft size and position.

Effect of meniscectomy

Meniscal tears cause pain and dysfunction and predispose the knee to articular cartilage degeneration. The size, location, and orientation of the tear will determine if a torn meniscus retains its biomechanical function [22]. Meniscus tears are repaired when possible, but partial and total meniscectomies are still necessary, causing altered biomechanics and detrimental effects that have been recognized for decades [30]. The relationship between meniscectomy and degenerative changes is clear [33–38], particularly in the lateral compartment where unique biomechanical and anatomic factors lead to a higher risk for degeneration than in the medial compartment [15,16,18,39]. Under physiologic conditions, the lateral meniscus carries most of the load in the lateral compartment, whereas the medial compartment shares the load almost equally between the meniscus and the exposed articular cartilage [16].

Historical perspective of meniscal allograft transplantation

The first human joint transplantations occurred a century ago [40,41], but the first true MAT occurred in 1972 when Zukor and colleagues [42] reported on a series of 33 fresh MATs. Size-matching a donor to a recipient within narrow time constraints because of primitive allograft processing techniques [43] cause logistical challenges such as scheduling surgery with short notice. MAT has gained popularity, as the development of safe and effective allograft tissue preservation and storage techniques has allowed for the creation of an inventory of variously sized menisci, and its protective effect on articular cartilage has been demonstrated in rabbits [44]. Graft preparation and sterilization methods have been refined to optimize healing and revascularization rates [11,45,46], graft shrinkage [47–49], cellularity [50,51], and donor and host DNA levels [52].

Immunogenicity

Animal studies have not demonstrated a predictable humeral or cellular-based immunologic rejection response from bone allografts in rabbits [53] or implanted meniscal allografts in goats [52,54] or mice [55].

The most immunogenic portions of the meniscal allograft are the cellular elements of the cancellous bone anchors [56], but studies of even massive bone allograft implantation [57] demonstrated a low rate of clinically meaningful immunogenic reactions. IL-17, which is a recently discovered pro-inflammatory family of cytokines secreted by activated T cells, seems to be operative in disparate tissues such as articular cartilage, bone, and meniscus and other soft tissues of the body, and to play a role in the homeostasis of these tissues in their healthy state [58]. Although meniscal allograft rejection has been reported [59], most series have not reported significant sequelae related to immunologic rejection. De Boer and Koudstaal [60] implanted a nontissue-antigen–matched cryopreserved meniscal allograft in the lateral compartment of a patient's knee that remained metabolically active with excellent clinical results and did not differ from control specimens. van Arkel and colleagues [61] and Khoury and colleagues [62] reported antibodies against the HLA complex [56] using nontissue-antigen–matched cryopreserved meniscal allografts without accompanying graft failure.

Graft procurement and processing

Because of difficulties harvesting and distributing fresh donor allografts to a size-matched recipient within a few days of harvest, fresh menisci suitable for allograft implantation have given way to bank-preserved meniscal allografts. Stringent donor screening include a comprehensive medical and social history as a critical first step in ensuring disease-free allograft tissue. The American Association of Tissue Banks has defined the recommended testing protocol [63]. Serologic screening is performed for HIV p24 antigen, HIV-1/HIV-2 antibody, human T-lymphotropic virus 1 and human T-lymphotropic

virus 2, hepatitis B surface antigen, hepatitis B core antibody, antibodies to hepatitis C virus, and syphilis. Most banks perform polymerase chain reaction (PCR) testing, which detects one HIV-infected cell out of 1 million cells. The current window of time for development of detectable antibodies to HIV is approximately 20 to 25 days (prior to that, a donor may be infected but test negative for HIV). Blood cultures for aerobic and anaerobic bacteria are conducted and lymph node sampling may be performed.

Graft processing, including debridement, ultrasonic/pulsatile washing, and use of ethanol to denature proteins, further lowers disease transmission risk. Freezing further lowers the risk, but HIV can survive washing, freezing, and freeze-drying [64]. Safety clearly depends on donor screening and not graft processing. The current risk for HIV transmission by frozen connective-tissue allografts is estimated to be 1 in 8 million [65].

The tissue is procured within 12 hours after death (fresh grafts) or within 24 hours after death if the body has been stored at 4°C. Currently, tissue may be harvested with the use of sterile surgical technique or it may be procured in a clean, nonsterile environment and secondarily sterilized. Harvested tissue is preserved by one of four methods: it can be fresh, cryopreserved, fresh-frozen, or lyophilized. Fresh and cryopreserved allografts contain viable cells, whereas fresh-frozen and lyophilized tissues are acellular at the time of transplantation. Fresh tissue is harvested under sterile conditions within 12 hours after death. The tissue is stored in a culture medium at 4°C or 37°C to maintain viable cells. Transplantation must be completed within several days of graft procurement, resulting in difficult logistics [66]. The exact rate and duration of cell viability is unknown. Jackson and colleagues [48] used DNA probes to demonstrate that all of the donor cells in a fresh meniscal transplant were rapidly replaced by host cells. Cryopreservation includes use of a cryoprotectant (ie, dimethylsulfoxide) to maintain cell viability and graft biomechanics [67]. Fresh-frozen grafts are rapidly frozen to −80°C, killing cells but maintaining material properties. Lyophilization, or freeze-drying, kills cells, affects graft material properties, and causes shrinkage [45,68]. Unlike fresh osteochondral grafts, the morphologic and biochemical characteristics of meniscal allografts do not depend heavily on cell viability. Therefore, the most commonly implanted grafts are either fresh-frozen or cryopreserved, and animal studies have shown no important differences between theses two methods [48,69].

Secondary sterilization with ethylene oxide, gamma irradiation, or chemical means may be used for fresh-frozen or lyophilized grafts. The amount of gamma irradiation required to eliminate viral DNA (at least 3.0 mrads [30,000 Gy]) may adversely affect the material properties of the meniscus [12]. Lower doses of gamma irradiation (<2.0 mrads [<20,000 Gy]) may be used for bacterial sterilization. Ethylene oxide is used only for lyophilized grafts, but it is not recommended because the ethylene chlorohydrin byproduct has been found to induce synovitis [70]. Chemical sterilization may be performed using proprietary bactericidal/virucidal solutions. In general, however, secondary sterilizing for meniscal allografts is not preferred.

Indications for meniscus transplantation

The ideal patient for meniscal allograft transplantation is a young but skeletally mature nonobese individual who has stable knee ligaments, normal anatomic alignment, and normal articular cartilage and is seeking treatment for pain in a meniscal deficient compartment. There must be no inflammatory arthritis, synovial disease, or history of infection in the involved knee. The patient should be too young for total knee arthroplasty. There is no upper chronologic age limit, but patients who have meniscal deficiencies and are in their mid-50s often have significant arthritis. Skeletal maturity is necessary to avoid causing asymmetric physeal arrest and progressive angular deformity.

To optimize the mechanical environment of the implanted meniscus, obesity should be a contraindication to meniscal transplantation. Untreated comorbidities of ligament instability, axial limb malalignment, and cartilage defects or degeneration also cause a hostile mechanical environment. These comorbidities can often be treated with simultaneous ligament reconstruction, osteotomy, or cartilage restoration. Even slight angular deviation compared with the contralateral limb may require an osteotomy. Concomitant or staged procedures is discussed later.

Fairbanks changes in meniscectomized knees range from the formation of an anteroposterior ridge projecting downward from the margin of the femoral condyle over the meniscal site to a generalized flattening of the marginal half of the femoral articular surface of the involved compartment, resulting in narrowing of the joint space on the involved side often associated with varus/valgus deformity of the knee [4]. Serious articular disease (ie, late grade III or IV) [71] and radiographic signs of flattening of the femoral condyle or marked osteophyte formation lead to poor graft survival, however, and are the most common contraindications to meniscal transplantation [72–74]. Restoration of the normal meniscal anatomy could decelerate or prevent degenerative change, but this is unproven. Systemic metabolic condition or local inflammatory condition affecting the knee is a contraindication to meniscal transplantation. Synovial disease or metabolic conditions will damage meniscal allografts. Immunodeficiency or a history of infection in the involved knee is a contraindication to meniscal transplantation, as the potential for devastating outcomes outweighs the potential for benefit of this procedure.

The surgeon must identify the specific motivation for a patient seeking transplantation and adjust expectations for partial, short-term pain relief. MAT could potentially retard osteoarthritis but it is primarily a pain-relieving effort. The patient should seek treatment for pain in the meniscal deficient compartment, and understand that at best, meniscal transplantation does not prevent the need for total knee arthroplasty.

Patient evaluation

After meniscectomy, patients report a gradual increase of joint-line pain, activity-related swelling, pain that changes with the ambient barometric pressure, and occasionally painful "giving-way" caused by quadriceps inhibition. A thorough history of the index injury and subsequent treatments, such as ligament reconstruction or management of articular cartilage lesions, are needed. Physical examination is essential to reveal malalignment, ligament deficiency, or articular cartilage lesions that would modify treatment plans. Patients generally have tenderness on the involved joint line often with a palpable osseous change at the femoral or tibial condyle. An effusion may or may not be present. For a patient to receive a transplant, range of motion must be normal.

Routine radiographs include weight-bearing anteroposterior view of both knees in full extension, a non–weight-bearing 45° flexion lateral view, and an axial view of the patellofemoral joint. A 45° flexion weight-bearing posteroanterior view can identify joint narrowing not seen on extension views [75]. Long-cassette mechanical axis films should be obtained if there is clinical malalignment. MRI techniques of two-dimensional fast spin-echo and three-dimensional fat suppression with and without intra-articular gadolinium can detail articular cartilage [76]. Three-phase bone scans are rarely used to detect increased uptake in the involved compartment.

Allograft sizing

The appropriate size of an absent meniscus cannot be determined by measuring the contralateral meniscus in the same compartment, as meniscal allografts are side- and compartment-specific, nor can the allograft size be predicted by a patient's height [77]. MRIs, radiographs, and CT scans have overestimated [78], underestimated [79], or in the case of CT arthrogram [74], over- and underestimated the size of meniscus allografts. Because of these potential inaccuracies, plain radiographs are most commonly used to size allografts [80,81]. Preoperatively, precise measurements are made on anteroposterior and lateral radiographs, with magnification markers placed on the skin at the level of the proximal part of the tibia. The surgeon should be familiar with the sizing techniques used by the tissue provider to minimize the chance of a size mismatch. Most commonly, the technique described by Pollard and colleagues [80] is used. The meniscal width is determined on an anteroposterior radiograph after correction for magnification. Meniscal length is calculated on the lateral radiograph on the basis of the sagittal length of the tibial plateau. Following correction for magnification, this length is multiplied by 0.8 for the medial meniscus and by 0.7 for the lateral meniscus. With use of this technique, size mismatch occurs less than 5% of the time. If the surgeon perioperatively judges the graft to be the incorrect size or compartment, the meniscus is not used. Small size mismatches can be handled with only minor modifications and are likely to have minimal effects on anatomic restoration, but accurate sizing is key to maximizing graft survival and chondroprotection [82].

Surgical techniques

Meniscal allograft transplantation replaces an absent or deficient meniscus in an anatomic position and restores the original meniscofemoral or meniscotibial articulation. The transplantation can be performed either open or with an arthroscopically assisted technique. The two methods have similar outcomes, but arthroscopic techniques are now routinely used because of the reduced surgical morbidity [45,72,83–89].

Meniscal allografts are anchored with either a bone bridge that rigidly fixes the distance between the anterior and posterior horns, or separate bone plugs on the anterior and posterior horns. For both techniques, the meniscus must be placed in an anatomic position with secure bone anchorage of the anterior and posterior horns [18,20,21]. The medial side may be anchored with either plugs or a bridge, whereas plugs are used only for medial transplants and not on the lateral side where the proximity to the anterior and posterior horns [90] risks tunnel communication. Using bone plugs on the medial side allows minor modifications to match the variable position of the anterior horn [77,91]. Proponents of a bone bridge on the medial side point out the ease of insertion and maintenance of the anatomic relationship between the allograft horns [86,92]. The decision to use a bridge or plugs on the medial side depends on surgeon preference.

Patient positioning and initial preparation

The patient is placed under general anesthesia and intravenous prophylactic antibiotics are administered. Before placing the patient in the desired leg holder, an examination under anesthesia is performed to confirm ligament stability. The patient is supine with the leg either unsupported with a lateral post placed just proximal to the knee, or placed in a midthigh leg holder with a tourniquet on but not inflated. The position of the leg holder should be proximal enough to allow ample exposure to the posterolateral and posteromedial corners for an inside-out meniscal repair, but distal enough to allow considerable valgus or varus stress to be placed on the knee without undue concern of a femur fracture. Standard arthroscopic portals are used and a diagnostic arthroscopy is performed to confirm the absence of significant chondral injuries in the recipient compartment, particularly if prior surgeries were performed by a different surgeon. The debridement of residual meniscal tissue should be performed without a tourniquet to verify a vascularized recipient meniscocapsular interface during debridement.

For both fixation techniques, the initial steps for medial and lateral meniscal transplantation are similar and are performed in the recipient compartment only. The host meniscus is debrided arthroscopically to a 1- to 2-mm peripheral rim until punctate bleeding occurs. A remnant of the anterior and posterior horns is left to clearly identify their location during tunnel creation (plugs) or slot formation (bridge). A low modified notchplasty on either the medial (protect posterior cruciate ligament [PCL]) or lateral (protect ACL) femoral condyle will facilitate allograft passage and visualization. A inside-out meniscal repair incision at the posterolateral or posteromedial corner is also used.

Bone plug technique

Separate bone plugs are often used to anchor the anterior and posterior horns of the medial meniscus. For this procedure, the involved compartment is prepared in the same manner as if performing a bridge technique. Two 9-mm cylindrical bone plugs are cored from the meniscal allograft, preserving all soft tissue attachment of the meniscal horns. No. 2 braided nonabsorbable polyethylene sutures are passed through 1.5-mm drill holes in each plug. The posterior horn bone plug can be undersized by 1 mm to facilitate passage and seating in the tunnel. A traction stitch in the posterior medial corner of the allograft will facilitate implantation (Fig. 1).

A modified low notchplasty between the fibers of the PCL and the medial femoral condyle will improve visualization and facilitate plug passage. To drill the recipient tunnels, an ACL tibial guide is used to pass a pin from the medial to the tibial tubercle to the exact center of the posterior horn, and reamed to 9 mm. The anterior horn is anterior to the footprint of the ACL at the anterior margin of the tibial plateau. The anterior tunnel is generally made after the meniscus is seated posteriorly and repaired peripherally with inside-out sutures.

Viewing from the lateral portal, the medial portal is expanded to receive the allograft. Next, the posteriomedial traction stitch is passed through the knee and out the posteromedial corner meniscus repair incision. The posterior bone plug stitch is then passed into the knee and out through the posterior horn tunnel using a suture passing device. Maintaining tension on the traction stitches at the posteromedial corner and posterior bone plug, a valgus stress is placed on the knee to open the medial compartment while the allograft is guided through the expanded

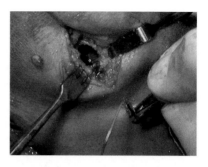

Fig. 2. The anterior horn plug is pulled into a blind-end tunnel at the anterior horn attachment with sutures passed through the anterior cortex.

medial portal and into the medial side of the joint. Positioning the bone plug in the posterior tunnel takes patience and persistence, but is facilitated by the low medial notchplasty and removal part of the medial tibial eminence, and by placing a valgus stress on the knee while pulling on the traction stitch with the knee positioned in about 30° of flexion. After the meniscus is reduced in the medial compartment, the knee is cycled several times to properly position the meniscus.

After the meniscus is secured posteriorly, the anterior horn bone plug is press-fit into a blind tunnel through the host anterior horn footprint. Sutures are passed through the anterior cortex of the proximal tibia with a free cutting needle and tied over bone (Fig. 2). This technique avoids an additional stress riser in the tibial metaphysis and does not interfere with a tibial ACL tunnel if a simultaneous ACL reconstruction is performed.

Eight to ten vertically placed 2-0 nonabsorbable mattress sutures are placed from posterior to anterior with use of a standard inside-out meniscal repair technique. On the medial side, all-inside bioabsorbable devices are a reasonable choice to secure the most posterior aspect of the meniscus to minimize the risk for neurovascular injury, but their pull-out strength is less than that of vertical sutures and they provide only single-point fixation [93,94].

Bridge in slot technique

Detailed descriptions of the bridge in slot technique are available elsewhere [85,86]. The slot is created directly in line with the anterior and posterior meniscal horns of the recipient compartment. A mini-arthrotomy is made either directly adjacent to the patellar tendon in line with the host anterior and posterior horns or by splitting the tendon. Arthro-

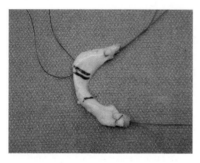

Fig. 1. Anchoring sutures are passed through each bone plug and a monofilament traction suture is placed into the posteromedial edge of the meniscus to facilitate reduction during implantation.

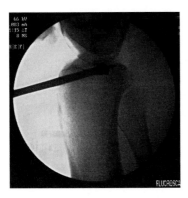

Fig. 3. Fluoroscopic lateral view is used to monitor location of reamer with respect to posterior tibia.

scopic electrocautery is used to mark a line between the centers of the horn footprints. Next, a 4-mm burr is used to create a superficial reference slot along this line. This reference slot should be the depth of the burr and should match the sagittal slope of the tibia. A depth gauge is placed into the slot and hooked onto the posterior tibia to confirm that it is of uniform height and depth, and to accurately measure the anteroposterior dimension of the slot. A drill guide chucked at the measured depth is used to insert a guide pin parallel to the tibial slope, taking care not to penetrate the posterior cortex of the tibial plateau. It is recommended that the guide wire placement and reaming be performed under fluoroscopic control (Fig. 3). The guide pin is advanced to but not through the posterior edge of the tibial plateau. An 8-mm cannulated reamer is advanced over the guide wire, and an 8 × 10-mm box cutter creates a slot. A rasp is used to assure uniformity in width and depth and

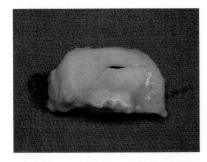

Fig. 4. The thawed lateral meniscal allograft is prepared on the back table simultaneously with trough preparation in the lateral tibial plateau of the recipient. The unprepared allograft is an en bloc section of the meniscus and the hemiplateau, incorporating the anterior and posterior horns.

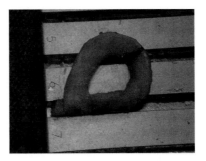

Fig. 5. The width of the lateral meniscus bridge measured carefully with the provided jig.

to prevent impingement of the prepared allograft bone bridge.

Allograft preparation

The allograft arrives from the tissue bank as a hemiplateau with the meniscus attached. All non-meniscal soft tissue is removed and the exact location of the anterior and posterior horn anchors are identified (Fig. 4). Using a cutting guide, the bridge is then cut to 7 × 10 mm. The authors recommend undersizing the full length of the bridge by 1 mm to facilitate passage through the slot. The prepared bridge is tested for ease of passage though calibrated troughs on the back table (Fig. 5). The posterior wall of the bridge should be flush or slanted slightly anterior to the fibers of the posterior horn attachment to allow for insertion at the most posterior edge of the prepared slot. Bone anterior to the anterior horn should be left in place to allow for safer graft manipulation during insertion. An 0-PDS vertical mattress traction suture is placed at the junction of the posterior and middle thirds (Fig. 6).

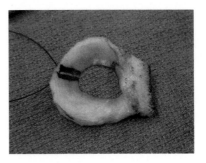

Fig. 6. The prepared bone bridge should have a minimal amount of bone posterior to the posterior horn insertion to avoid impingement leading to improper position of the posterior horn.

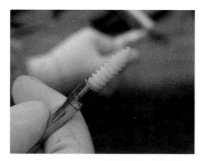

Fig. 7. An interference screw machined from allograft bone is used for fixation of the bone bridge in the slot.

To insert the graft, the traction sutures in the allograft are shuttled through the posterior incision using zone-specific meniscus repair cannulae. The allograft is inserted though the arthrotomy and aligned with the slot as the meniscus is reduced under the femoral condyle by pulling on the traction suture and cycling the knee to allow the femoral condyle to engage and position the allograft meniscus. Simultaneous varus or valgus stress will open the recipient compartment. The slightly undersized meniscal bone bridge allows the meniscus to achieve its proper position by sliding freely within the tibial slot. Once the proper bone-bridge position is achieved, a guide wire is inserted between the bone bridge and the more midline wall of the slot. A tap is used over the guide wire to create a path for an interference screw with the bone bridge held firmly in place by an elevator placed through the arthrotomy. A 7 × 20-mm or 8 × 20-mm bioabsorbable interference screw is inserted while maintaining meticulous rotational control of the bone bridge. Of particular importance is the fixation of the allograft bone bridge within the host tibial slot to maintain the proper anatomic position of the meniscal horns. There has been recent success with allograft interference screws created from cortical allograft bone (Fig. 7) [86]. However, bioabsorbable screws offer an acceptable alternative.

The final arthroscopic examination of the implanted allograft should confirm not only that the graft is anatomically reduced under the condyle but also that the proper size was selected. The lack of undulation on the surface indicates that the tissue is not distorted in situ (Fig. 8). The meniscus is then sutured as described in the bone plug technique.

Combined procedures

It is often advisable to perform simultaneous or staged procedures to treat comorbidities that may

coexist in the setting of meniscal transplantation. Limb axis malalignment, ligament instability, or cartilage defects may require an osteotomy, ligament reconstruction, or a cartilage resurfacing procedure. When combining a meniscus transplant with other procedures, it is important to plan the exact sequence of events in a detailed pre-operative plan.

Corrective osteotomy

If the recipient compartment is under more than physiologic compression, realignment osteotomy should be performed as an adjunct procedure [95]. In the setting of medial meniscal deficiency and varus alignment, a combined meniscus transplantation and high tibial osteotomy should be performed. In contrast to a standard high tibial osteotomy for isolated medical compartment osteoarthritis, in which the aim is to correct the mechanical axis laterally to 66% of the width of the tibial plateau in the lateral compartment [96], high tibial osteotomies combined with medial meniscus should correct the mechanical axis to just beyond neutral. The authors recommend the use of an opening medial osteotomy to create a valgus correction, but the more traditional closing lateral osteotomy is also a reasonable option. Commercially available instrumentation (Arthrex, Naples, Florida) allows for a technically precise, simple, rapidly performed opening medial osteotomy with rigid fixation. In the less-common scenario of valgus angulation of a knee joint with lateral compartment disease, a distal femoral osteotomy is advisable. Generally the authors recommend an opening lateral distal femoral osteotomy with rigid plate fixation, although other techniques and fixation methods

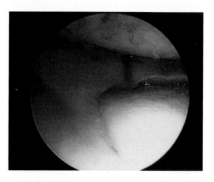

Fig. 8. Proper position, size, and suturing of the allograft under femoral condyle is evinced by the smooth contour in situ without undulations.

have been described, including a percutaneous dome osteotomy combined with temporary external fixation and intramedullary nail fixation [97]. For varus and valgus osteotomies, care must be taken not to overcorrect.

When performing a high tibial osteotomy with MAT, the bridge and slot technique will prevent communication of metaphyseal tunnels with the osteotomy. If bone plugs are used, the tunnels should exit as far proximal as possible to avoid traversing the osteotomy. Arthroscopic evaluation, soft-tissue preparation, notchplasty, and slot or tunnel creation of the meniscal transplant technique are performed before the osteotomy. Osteotomies should be performed as far distally as possible, and secure fixation of the osteotomy must withstand the valgus stress required for graft insertion and meniscal repair. Inserting osteotomy fixation hardware under fluoroscopic guidance is important to direct screws away from the meniscal tunnels or trough.

Meniscal allograft transplantation and anterior cruciate ligament reconstruction

Uncorrected ligamentous instability is a contraindication to meniscal transplantation. A preoperative evaluation of a meniscal-deficient knee includes a careful analysis of the ligamentous instability. This evaluation includes the history of injury, a familiarity with previous surgical procedures, MRI and radiograph information, and ideally, an arthrometric evaluation. An examination of the ACL under anesthesia is more reliable than while the patient is awake. Ideally, if a patient had prior surgeries, documentation of that exam would be available from those previous surgeries.

The biomechanical interdependence between an ACL reconstruction and the presence or condition of functional menisci is well documented [98]. A successful ACL reconstruction relies on an intact medial meniscus to minimize anterior-posterior stress [10,39], and an intact ACL, in turn, protects menisci and articular cartilage [99,100]. Simultaneous meniscus transplantation and ACL reconstruction have been shown to be mutually beneficial in properly selected patients [101,102].

If a meniscus transplant is combined with either primary or revision ACL, there are several issues to consider related to the three-dimensional relationship of tunnels in the tibial metaphysis. Prior tunnel expansion and position and intended locations of new tunnels (in the setting of revision ACL reconstruc-

tion), ACL graft selection, and meniscus anchor method offer variability to address the needs of each particular patient. With bone plug technique, all soft-tissue and osseous portions of the meniscal transplant technique are performed first. The tibial tunnel for the anterior cruciate reconstruction is then drilled slightly more medially than usual to avoid confluence between it and the tunnel for the posterior horn of the meniscus. The remaining portions of the anterior cruciate reconstruction are performed as usual. With a bone-bridge technique, the tibial tunnel for the anterior cruciate reconstruction is reamed after placement of the meniscal allograft. Placing the tunnel entrance slightly distally and medially on the tibia can minimize confluence between the tunnel and the lateral slot. The meniscal bone bridge may, however, be partially intersected without untoward effects during creation of the tibial tunnel [101]. Use of a hamstring graft for the reconstruction of the ACL may facilitate graft passage by allowing for a smaller-diameter tibial ACL tunnel.

Occasionally, patients have combined varus alignment, ACL deficiency, and an absent medial meniscus with intact articular cartilage. These patients are typically managed with reconstruction of the ACL at the time of a high tibial osteotomy. The meniscal transplantation is performed simultaneously with these procedures only in rare situations, such as in very young patients. More commonly, meniscal allograft reconstruction is performed in a delayed fashion in a patient who has persistent symptoms following recovery from the initial procedures.

Meniscal allograft transplantation and cartilage restoration procedures

When combining cartilage restoration with meniscal transplantation in the same compartment, it is important to plan the exact sequence of events in a detailed preoperative plan. It is typically easier and safer for chondral procedures to be performed after all steps of the meniscal transplant have been completed to avoid inadvertent damage to the periosteal patch or osteochondral graft during meniscal instrumentation or suture repair [92]. On the other hand, the anterior horn of the transplanted meniscus could be damaged by subsequent cartilage procedure on the ipsilateral femoral condyle. For example, implanting an osteochondral allograft and performing a meniscal transplant will require that the posterior horn anchor be established before preparing the articular cartilage defect and implanting the osteochondral allograft

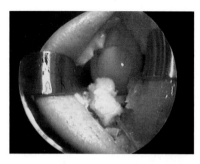

Fig. 9. Osteochondral allograft and simultaneous meniscus allograft transplantation in the same compartment requires carefully sequenced steps to avoid damaging either allograft.

plug. The bone plug and anterior horn of the meniscal allograft are gently retracted out of harms way during implantation of the osteochondral graft and inserted in a blind tunnel at the anatomic site of the anterior horn after the osteochondral graft implantation is completed (Fig. 9).

Outcomes

The literature supports good to excellent results of roughly 85% following MAT, with a measurable decrease in pain and increase in activity level, provided there is proper patient selection. There is a greater risk for graft failure in irradiated grafts, uncorrected malalignment, osteoarthritic compartments, and absence of bone anchorage of the allograft [103]. There is not a clear correlation with graft shrinkage or decreased cellular viability and poorer outcomes. There is a trend toward better results in more recent series, which reflects a collective improvement in patient selection, graft processing, and surgical technique over the last 15 years.

There is not a clear correlation with the physical appearance of the graft and outcome. In 1989, Milachowski and colleagues [45] reported that of six fresh-frozen and 16 freeze-dried meniscus allografts, the fresh-frozen grafts had a more normal gross appearance than the freeze-dried grafts that demonstrated more shrinkage, but this did not correlate with poorer outcomes. In 1999, Carter's [84] second-look arthroscopy of 38 cases at 2 years demonstrated four that had visible shrinkage of the graft and two that had progression of arthritis. These patients had inferior results. In contrast, Stollsteimer and colleagues [88] reported substantial pain relief in all 23 patients following cryopreserved allografts despite an average shrinkage of 37% found on MRI.

A decrease in cellularity and viability of the meniscus tissue has not correlated directly with poorer outcomes. In 1996, Wilcox and Goble [31] reported that 17 of 18 patients (94%) had a significant decrease in knee pain and improvement in function with universal patient satisfaction [71]. A second-look arthroscopy was performed on 13 patients (13 grafts) of which ten (71%) had a well-healed and functional meniscus. Biopsy performed on 8 of 14 grafts revealed an average of 80% viable meniscal tissue. A year earlier, van Arkel and de Boer [89] reported their prospective outcomes of 23 patients following cryopreserved meniscal transplant, of which 20 (87%) reported successful results, and peripheral healing was demonstrated in all but three of the patients examined with second-look arthroscopy. Histologic analysis demonstrated revascularization with viable meniscal chondrocytes. The three patients who failed had uncorrected malalignment. In 2001, Rath and colleagues [104] reported that 8 of 22 cryopreserved menisci (36%) tore after 2 years, necessitating six partial and two total meniscectomies and reimplantation, and the removed tissue revealed reduced cellularity compared with normal or torn native menisci. Fourteen patients reported a successful result, but there is no information regarding the cellularity of these more successful grafts.

Articular cartilage degeneration or a lack of allograft bone anchorage correlates with poor outcomes. In 1993, Garrett [72] reported that 35 of 43 (81%) patients were asymptomatic 2 years after complex procedures, with most failures occurring in knees that had grade IV chondromalacia. In 1994, Shelton and Dukes [105] reported that 15 of 16 patients who had less than grade II arthritic changes reported a significant decrease in pain and no recurrent effusion, whereas four patients who had transplantations into degenerative compartments had only slight improvement in symptoms. All second-look arthroscopies demonstrated complete peripheral healing, however, and although there was an average shrinkage of 15%, cellular viability was confirmed by biopsy. In 1995, Noyes and Barber-Westin [103] reported on 96 irradiated grafts, many of which were secured with bone at the posterior horn, but none had bone anchorage in the anterior and posterior horns. In this series, 29 menisci were removed by 2 years. Only 9% of the grafts healed, 31% were partially healed, and 58% failed clinically, with higher rates of failure in knees with arthrosis ($P < .001$) at a rate of 50% failure in knees with grade IV arthrosis. In 2001, Rodeo and colleagues [106,107] reported successful results in 22 of 33 (67%) patients. Of these, 14 of the 16 (88%) transplants that were anchored to bone at the anterior and posterior horns had good results, whereas only 8 of the 17 (47%) nonbone anchorage transplants were successful. In contrast to these studies, however, Cameron and Saha [83] reported good to excellent results in 87% of 67 irradiated allografts without bone anchors, many in patients who had advanced unicompartmental arthritis.

Several series have demonstrated the benefit of combining procedures to treat comorbid conditions that would otherwise be contraindications to MAT. Ligament reconstruction and cartilage restoration procedures can optimize the mechanical environment for the meniscal allograft. MAT can, in turn, provide protection for ligament reconstruction or cartilage restoration procedures. Zukor and colleagues [42] combined fresh meniscal and osteochondral allografts for knee injuries resulting in focal chondral defects and a deficient meniscus. At 1 year, 26 of 33 patients (79%) were clinically successful, with no meniscal failures. In the series by Veltri and colleagues [74] of 16 deep frozen or cryopreserved meniscal transplantations, 11 of which underwent either ACL or PCL reconstruction at surgery, 85% were asymptomatic. Sekiya and colleagues [108] reported retrospectively that 24 of 28 (86%) patients who had undergone ACL reconstruction with meniscal transplantation had normal or nearly normal IKDC scores, and nearly 90% had a normal or nearly normal Lachman and pivot shift exam, with an average maximum manual KT arthrometer side-to-side difference of 1.5 mm. Joint-space narrowing of the transplanted compartments was not significantly different from that of the contralateral knee. From these results the investigators concluded that restoration of meniscal function combined with ACL reconstruction may provide protection for the articular cartilage and improve joint stability, thereby eliminating a contraindication for meniscal transplantation. Yoldas and colleagues [102] reported on 31 patients following meniscus transplantation with and without combined ACL reconstruction. In this group, 20 patients received meniscal transplantation and ACL reconstruction and 11 patients who had stable ligaments underwent meniscal transplantation alone. Both groups had MAT with bone plugs medially and a bone bridge laterally. There were no significant differences in knee scores or joint-space narrowing on flexion weight-bearing views based on medial or lateral meniscus, concurrent ACL reconstruction, or the degree of chondrosis at arthroscopy. KT-1000 arthrometry revealed an average side-to-side difference of 2 mm (range, 2–7 mm). MAT with ligament reconstruction or cartilage restoration can provide relief of symptoms and restore high levels of function.

Discussion

Meniscus deficiency is considered by some authors to be a greatly underestimated problem in orthopedics today [103]. To patients, meniscal deficiency is a problem leading to pain, swelling, arthritic changes, and limitation of activity. To physicians, meniscal deficiency is a problem because of the lack of suitable solutions for their patients. To society, the sequelae of a meniscus-deficient knee translate into a loss of productivity and an increase in monetary expenditures for health care benefits. Many patient- and surgeon-specific variables, such as the degree of arthrosis, method of graft processing, surgical technique, types of concomitant procedures, and method of evaluation, differ among studies. Thus, it is difficult to make comparisons or draw conclusions on the basis of the existing literature.

The average age of the patient who is affected by knee ligament instability is 21 years. The average age of the patient who undergoes a total knee arthroplasty is 70 years. The average age for MAT is 33 years [109]. Knee instability primarily disables young athletes. Knees requiring salvage procedures, such as total knee arthroplasties, primarily affect individuals who are retirement-age, whereas patients who have meniscal-deficient knees represent a greater percentage of individuals within the day-to-day work force and who have major responsibilities in their personal lives. It should, therefore, be medically understandable that even a documented short-term improvement in an otherwise disabled population could be defined as a success.

Obtaining secure bone anchorage of the anterior and posterior horns, although technically more demanding, is necessary to maximize the potential for a successful outcome. The series by Rodeo [106], in which overall there were only 22 (66%) of 33 successful outcomes, demonstrated a much higher rate, with 14 (88%) successful outcomes of the 16 patients who had obtained bone anchorage compared with only 8 (47%) of the 17 patients who did not obtain bone anchorage. These clinical results coincide with the biomechanical understanding of the potential for benefit of a meniscal allograft [18,21,32].

The degree of arthrosis at the time of allograft transplantation is possibly the most important factor predicting outcome, with advanced arthrosis associated with the highest failure rates [89,103,110]. Using MRI, Rodeo [106] demonstrated that knees with advanced arthrosis had a greater propensity for graft extrusion, a finding believed to be associated with an increased risk for failure. Correcting limb malalignment is another factor believed to be critical for success [83]. van Arkel and de Boer [89] attributed their three graft failures to uncorrected limb alignment. Cameron and Saha [83] performed osteotomy in 34 of 63 patients. By realigning the knees to "unload" the involved compartment, they achieved a success rate comparable with that in the group as a whole, with a good or excellent result in 85% or 87%, respectively.

Meniscal shrinkage rating is inaccurate. At second-look arthroscopy in 22 cases, Carter [84] believed only three showed size reduction. Milachowski and colleagues [45] noted shrinkage of 33% to 66% in 14 of 23 menisci examined by second-look arthroscopy. It is not known if shrinkage occurs because of a subclinical immune response with graft-remodeling during cellular repopulation, a poor quality graft, excessive graft-loading during healing, the surgical technique, knee arthrosis, or some variable not currently recognized. The study by Stollsteimer and colleagues [88] suggests a low correlation between graft shrinkage and symptoms, however. MRI scans have demonstrated that the grafts can look similar to a normal meniscus, whereas others have shown signals consistent with degenerative changes [84,88,103,107]. Second-look arthroscopy is often necessary to define the exact quality of graft-healing [111–114].

Whether meniscal grafts prevent the progression of arthritis is unknown. Rath and colleagues [104] reported that the compartment space of the involved knees of 11 patients averaged 5.2 mm before surgery and 4.5 mm 2 years after transplantation. Carter [84] reported 2 of 46 knees with radiographic progression at almost 3 years. Rabbit studies demonstrate equal rates of radiographic degenerative changes at 1 year in meniscectomized and transplanted animals [115].

With respect to combined procedures, uncorrected comorbidities are contraindications to meniscal transplantation, but the beneficial effect of combined procedures is emerging and the synergy of concomitant reconstructions is evident. When a cartilage restoration or ligament reconstruction protects a meniscal transplant, a mutually beneficial relationship exists between the healthy functioning meniscus transplant and the ligament reconstruction or cartilage resurfacing procedures.

Summary

Despite encouraging intermediate-term benefits, the true long-term function of the transplanted meniscus remains unknown. The transplant appears to remodel and experience changes in its collagen fiber architecture that affect its load-sharing capabilities and long-term survival. The meniscal transplant surgeon should advise patients that this procedure is indicated for patients who have few other options, and the procedure is likely not curative in the long-term. However, establishing a pain-free and mechanically stable environment for even an intermediate period of time (ie, 5 or 10 years), as supported by the literature, seems entirely justified given the lack of alternatives and the added benefit of placing a patient chronologically at an age more appropriate for arthroplasty should it become necessary.

References

[1] Mow VC, Ratcliff A, Chern KY, et al. Structure and function relationships of the meniscus and knee. In: Mow VC, Arnoczky SP, Jackson DW, editors. Knee meniscus: basic and clinical foundations. New York: Raven Press; 1992. p. 37.
[2] Elliott DM, Guilak F, Vail TP, et al. Tensile properties of articular cartilage are altered by meniscectomy in a canine model of osteoarthritis. J Orthop Res 1999; 17(4):503–8.
[3] MacConaill MA. The movements of bones and joints; the mechanical structure of articulating cartilage. J Bone Joint Surg Br 1951;33B(2):251–7.
[4] Fu FH, Thompson WO. Motion of the meniscus during knee flexion. In: Mow VC, Arnoczky SP, Jackson DW, editors. Knee meniscus: basic and clinical foundations. New York: Raven Press; 1992. p. 75.
[5] Levy IM, Torzilli PA, Warren RF. The effect of medial meniscectomy on anterior-posterior motion of the knee. J Bone Joint Surg Am 1982;64(6): 883–8.
[6] Shoemaker SC, Markolf KL. The role of the meniscus in the anterior-posterior stability of the loaded anterior cruciate-deficient knee. Effects of partial versus total excision. J Bone Joint Surg Am 1986;68(1): 71–9.
[7] Levy IM, Torzilli PA, Fisch ID. The contribution of the menisci to the stability of the knee. In: Mow VC, Arnoczky SP, Jackson DW, editors. Knee meniscus: basic and clinical foundations. New York: Raven Press; 1992. p. 107–15.
[8] Thompson WO, Thaette FL, Fu FH, et al. Tibial meniscal dynamics using three-dimensional reconstruction of magnetic resonance images. Am J Sports Med 1991;19:210–5.
[9] Jager A, Welsch F, Braune C, et al. Ten year follow-up after single incision anterior cruciate ligament reconstruction using patellar tendon autograft. Z Orthop Ihre Grenzgeb 2003;141(1):42–7.
[10] Shelbourne KD, Gray T. Results of anterior cruciate ligament reconstruction based on meniscus and

articular cartilage status at the time of surgery. Five-to fifteen-year evaluations. Am J Sports Med 2000; 28(4):446–52.

[11] Weismeier K, Worth CJ, Milachowski KA. [Transplantation of the meniscus. Experimental study.] Rev Chir Orthop Reparatrice Appar Mot 1988;74:155–9 [in French].

[12] Hsu RWW, Himeno S, Coventry MB. Transactions of the 34th Annual Meeting of the Orthopedic Research Society, vol. 13. Park Ridge (IL): Orthopedic Research Society; 1988.

[13] Rohrie H, Scholten R. Joint forces in the human pelvis-leg skeleton during walking. J Biomech 1984; 17(6):409–24.

[14] Ahmed AM. The load bearing of the knee meniscus. In: Mow VC, Arnoczky SP, Jackson DW, editors. Knee meniscus: basic and clinical foundations. New York: Raven Press; 1992. p. 59–73.

[15] Ahmed AM, Burke DL. In-vitro measurement of static pressure distribution in synovial joints–Part I: tibial surface of the knee. J Biomech Eng 1983; 105(3):216–25.

[16] Walker BF, Erkman MJ. The role of the menisci in force transmission across the knee. Clin Orthop 1975;(109):184–92.

[17] Baratz ME, Fu FH, Mengato R. Meniscal tears: the effect of meniscectomy and of repair on intra-articular contact areas and stress in the human knee. A preliminary report. Am J Sports Med 1986;14(4): 270–5.

[18] Paletta Jr GA, Manning T, Snell E, et al. The effect of allograft meniscal replacement on intraarticular contact area and pressures in the human knee. A biomechanical study. Am J Sports Med 1997;25(5): 692–8.

[19] Seedhom BB, Hargreaves DJ. Transmission of load in the knee joint with special reference to the role of the menisci, part II: experimental results, discussions, and conclusions. Eng Med 1979;8: 220–8.

[20] Alhalki MM, Howell SM, Hull ML. How three methods for fixing a medial meniscal autograft affect tibial contact mechanics. Am J Sports Med 1999;27: 320–8.

[21] Chen MI, Branch TP, Hutton WC. Is it important to secure the horns during lateral meniscal transplantation? A cadaveric study. Arthroscopy 1996;12(2): 174–81.

[22] DeHaven KE. [Meniscus resection versus reattachment of the meniscus.] Orthopade 1994;23:133–6 [in German].

[23] Szomor ZL, Martin TE, Bonar F, et al. The protective effects of meniscal transplantation on cartilage. An experimental study in sheep. J Bone Joint Surg Am 2000;82(1):80–8.

[24] Arnoczky SP, McDevitt CA. The meniscus: structure function, repair and replacement. In: Buckwalter JA, Einhorn TA, Simon SR, editors. Orthopedic basic Science: biology and biomechanics of the musculo-skeletal system. Rosemont (IL): American Academy of Orthopedic Surgeons; 2000. p. 531–45.

[25] Mow VC, Holmes MH, Lai WM. Fluid transport and mechanical properties of articular cartilage: a review. J Biomech 1984;17(5):377–94.

[26] Favenesi JA, Shaffer JC, Mow VC. Biphasic mechanical properties of knee meniscus. Trans Orthop Res Soc 1983;8:57.

[27] Fithian DC, Kelly MA, Mow VC. Material properties and structure-function relationships in the menisci. Clin Orthop Relat Res 1990;Mar(252):19–31.

[28] Skaggs DL, Warden WH, Mow VC. Radial tie fibers influence the tensile properties of the bovine medial meniscus. J Orthop Res 1994;12:176.

[29] Lee SJ, Aadalen KJ, Lorenz EP, et al. Tibiofemoral contact mechanics following serial medial meniscectomies in the human cadaveric knee, AOSSM Annual Meeting, Quebec City, June 24–27, 2004.

[30] Fairbank TJ. Knee joint changes after meniscectomy. J Bone Joint Surg Br 1948;30:664–70.

[31] Wilcox TR, Goble EM. Goble technique of meniscus transplantation. Am J Knee Surg 1996;9:1.

[32] Alhalki MM, Hull ML, Howell SM. Contact mechanics of the medial tibial plateau after implantation of a medial meniscal allograft. A human cadaveric study. Am J Sports Med 2000;28(3):370–6.

[33] Huckle JR. Is meniscectomy a benign procedure? A long-term follow-up study. Can J Surg 1965;8:254.

[34] Johnson RJ, Kettlekamp DB, Clark W, et al. Factors affecting late results after meniscectomy. J Bone Joint Surg Am 1974;56:719.

[35] Lynch MA, Henning CE. Osteoarthritis in the ACL deficient knee. In: Feagin Jr JA, editor. The cruciate ligaments. New York: Churchill, Livingstone; 1988. p. 385.

[36] Lynch MA, Henning CE, Glick KR. Knee joint surface changes: Long-term follow-up meniscus tear treatment and stable anterior cruciate ligament reconstruction. Clin Orthop 1983;172:148.

[37] O'Brien WR. Degenerative arthritis of the knee following anterior cruciate ligament injury: Role of the meniscus. Sports Med Arthroscopy Rev 1993; 1:114.

[38] Tapper EM, Hoover NW. Late results after meniscectomy. J Bone Joint Surg Am 1969;51(3):517–26.

[39] Levy IM, Torzilli PA, Gould JD, et al. The effect of lateral meniscectomy on motion of the knee. J Bone Joint Surg Am 1989;71(3):401–6.

[40] Lexer E. Substitution of whole or half Joints from freshly amputated extremities by free plastic operation. Surg Gynecol Obstet 1908;6:601–7.

[41] Lexer E. Joint transplantations and arthroplasty. Surg Gynecol Obstet 1925;40:782–809.

[42] Zukor DJ, Cameron JC, Brooks PJ, et al. The fate of human meniscal allografts. In: Ewing JW, editor. Articular cartilage and knee joint function: basic science and arthroscopy. New York: Raven Press; 1990. p. 147.

[43] Brown KL, Cruess RL. Bone and cartilage trans-

plantation in orthopedic surgery review. J Bone Joint Surg Am 1982;64:270.

[44] Cummins JF, Mansour JN, Howe Z, et al. Meniscal transplantation and degenerative articular change: An experimental study in the rabbit. Arthroscopy 1997; 13:485.

[45] Milachowski KA, Weismeier K, Worth CJ, et al. Homologous meniscus transplantation: Experimental and clinical results. Int Orthop 1989;13:1–11.

[46] Milachowski KA, Kohn D, Wirth CJ. Transplantation of allogenic menisci. Orthopade 1994; 23:160.

[47] Arnoczky SB, O'Brian S, DeCarlo E, et al. Cell survival after transplantation of fresh meniscal allograft: DNA probe analysis in goat model. Am J Sports Med 1988;21:540.

[48] Jackson DW, Whelan J, Simon TM. Cell survival of the transplantation of fresh meniscal allograft: DNA probe analysis in a goat model. Am J Sports Med 1993;21:540–50.

[49] Mikic ZD, Brankoy MZ, Tubic MV, et al. Allograft meniscal transplantation in a dog. Acta Orthop Scand 1993;64:329.

[50] Arnoczky SP, McDevitt CA. Meniscal replacement using cryopreserved allograft: Experimental study in the dog. Clin Orthop 1990;252:121.

[51] Arnoczky SP, Milachowski KA. Meniscal allografts: where do we stand? In: Ewing JW, editor. Articular cartilage and the knee joint function: basic science and arthroscopy. New York: Raven Press; 1990. p. 129.

[52] Jackson DW, McDevitt CA, Simon TM, et al. Meniscal transplantation using fresh and cryo-preserved allograft: An experimental study in goats. Am J Sports Med 1992;20:646.

[53] Friedlaender GE, Strong DM, Sell KW. Studies on the antigenicity of bone. I. Freeze-dried and deep-frozen bone allografts in rabbits. J Bone Joint Surg Am 1976;58:854–8.

[54] Fabbriciani C, Lucania L. Meniscal allografts: Cryopreservation vs. deep frozen technique. An experimental study in goats. Knee Surg Sports Traumatol Arthrosc 1997;5:124.

[55] Ochi M, Ishida O, Daisaku H, et al. Immune response to fresh meniscal allografts in mice. J Surg Res 1995; 58(5):478–84.

[56] Goble EM, Kohn D, Verdonk R, et al. Meniscal substitutes—human experience. Scand J Med Sci Sports 1999;9:146–57.

[57] Friedlaender GE, Strong DM, Sell KW. Studies on the antigenicity of bone. II. Donor-specific anti-HLA antibodies in human recipients of freeze-dried allografts. J Bone Joint Surg Am 1984;66(1):107–12.

[58] Moseley TA, Haudenschild DR, Rose L, et al. Interleukin-17 family and IL-17 receptors. Cytokine Growth Factor Rev 2003;14(2):155–74.

[59] Hamlet W, Liu SH, Yang R. Destruction of a cyropreserved meniscal allograft: a case for acute rejection. Arthroscopy 1997;13(4):517–21.

[60] De Boer HH, Koudstaal J. The fate of meniscus cartilage after transplantation of cryopreserved non-tissue-antigen-matched allograft. A case report. Clin Orthop 1991;(266):145–51.

[61] van Arkel ER, van den Berg-Loonen EM, van Wersch JW, et al. Human leukocyte antigen sensitization after cryopreserved human meniscal transplantations. Transplantation 1997;64:531–3.

[62] Khoury MA, Goldberg VM, Stevenson S. Demonstration of HLA and ABH antigens in fresh and frozen human menisci by immunohistochemistry. J Orthop Res 1994;12(6):751–7.

[63] Standards for tissue banking. Mclean (VA): American Association of Tissue Banks; 2002.

[64] Nemzek JA, Arnoczky SP, Swenson CL. Retroviral transmission by the transplantation of connective-tissue allografts. An experimental study. J Bone Joint Surg Am 1994;76:1036–41.

[65] Buck BE, Resnick L, Shah SM, et al. Human immunodeficiency virus cultured from bone. Implications for transplantation. Clin Orthop 1990;251:249–53.

[66] Verdonk R, Van Daele P, Claus B, et al. Viable meniscus transplantation. Orthopade 1994;23: 153–9 [German].

[67] Arnoczky SP, McDevitt CA, Schmidt MB, et al. The effect of cryopreservation on canine menisci: a biochemical, morphologic, and biomechanical evaluation. J Orthop Res 1988;6:1–12.

[68] Yahia LH, Drouin G, Zukor D. The irradiation effect on the initial mechanical properties of meniscal grafts. Biomed Mater Eng 1993;3:211–21.

[69] Fabbriciani C, Lucania L, Milano G, et al. Meniscal allografts: cryopreservation vs deep-frozen technique. An experimental study in goats. Knee Surg Sports Traumatol Arthrosc 1997;5:124–34.

[70] Jackson DW, Windler GE, Simon TM. Intraarticular reaction associated with the use of freezedried, ethylene oxide-sterilized bone-patella tendon-bone allografts in the reconstruction of the anterior cruciate ligament. Am J Sports Med 1990;18:1–10.

[71] Outerbridge RE. The etiology of chondromalacia patellae. J Bone Joint Surg Br 1961;43:752–7.

[72] Garrett JC. Meniscal transplantation: review of forty-three cases with two-to-seven year follow up. Sports Med Arthroscopy Rev 1993;1:164–7.

[73] Siegel MG, Roberts CS. Meniscal allografts. Clin Sports Med 1993;12:59.

[74] Veltri DM, Warren RF, Wickiewicz TL, et al. Current status of allograft meniscal transplantation. Clin Orthop 1994;303:44.

[75] Rosenberg TD, Paulos LE, Parker RD, et al. The forty-five-degree posteroanterior flexion weight-bearing radiograph of the knee. J Bone Joint Surg Am 1988; 70:1479–83.

[76] Potter HG, Linklater JM, Allen AA, et al. Magnetic resonance imaging of articular cartilage in the knee. An evaluation with use of fast-spin-echo imaging. J Bone Joint Surg Am 1998;80:1276–84.

[77] Kohn D, Moreno B. Meniscus insertion anatomy

as a basis for meniscus replacement: a morphological cadaveric study. Arthroscopy 1995;11:96–103.

[78] Kennedy S, Shaffer B, Yao L. Preoperative planning in meniscal allograft reconstruction. Presented at the 24th annual meeting of the American Orthopedic Society for Sports Medicine. Orlando, FL, July 12, 1998.

[79] Carpenter JE, Wojtys EM, Huston LJ. Pre-operative sizing of meniscal replacements. Presented at the 12th annual meeting of the Arthroscopy Association of North America. Palm Desert, CA, April 1, 1993.

[80] Pollard ME, Kang Q, Berg EE. Radiographic sizing for meniscal transplantation. Arthroscopy 1995;11: 684–7.

[81] Shaffer B, Kennedy S, Klimkiewicz J, et al. Preoperative sizing of meniscal allografts in meniscus transplantation. Am J Sports Med 2000;28:524–33.

[82] Verdonk R, Kohn D. Harvest and conservation of meniscal allografts. Scand J Med Sci Sports 1999;9: 158–9.

[83] Cameron JC, Saha S. Meniscal allograft transplantation for unicompartmental arthritis of the knee. Clin Orthop 1997;337:164–71.

[84] Carter TR. Meniscal Allograft Transplantation. Sports Med Arthroscopy Rev 1999;7:51–62.

[85] Cole BJ, Fox JA, Lee SJ, et al. Bone bridge in slot technique for meniscal transplantation. Op Tech Sports Med 2003;11:144–55.

[86] Farr J, Meneghini RM, Cole BJ. Allograft interference screw fixation in meniscus transplantation. Arthroscopy 2004;20:322–7.

[87] Fox JA, Lee SJ, Cole BJ. Bone plug technique for meniscal transplantation. Op Tech Sports Med 2003;11:161–9.

[88] Stollsteimer GT, Shelton WR, Dukes A, et al. Meniscal allograft transplantation: a 1- to 5-year follow-up of 22 patients. Arthroscopy 2000;16:343–7.

[89] van Arkel ER, de Boer HH. Human meniscal transplantation. Preliminary results at 2 to 5-year follow-up. J Bone Joint Surg Br 1995;77(4):589–95.

[90] Johnson DL, Swenson TM, Livesay GA, et al. Insertion-site anatomy of the human menisci: gross, arthroscopic, and topographical anatomy as a basis for meniscal transplantation. Arthroscopy 1995;11: 386–94.

[91] Berlet GC, Fowler PJ. The anterior horn of the medial meniscus. An anatomic study of its insertion. Am J Sports Med 1998;26:540–3.

[92] Albrecht-Olsen P, Lind T, Kristensen G, et al. Failure strength of a new meniscus arrow repair technique: biomechanical comparison with horizontal suture. Arthroscopy 1997;13:183–7.

[93] Albrecht-Olsen P, Lind T, Kristensen G, et al. Failure strength of a new meniscus arrow repair technique: biomechanical comparison with horizontal suture. Arthroscopy 1997;13:183–7.

[94] Boenisch UW, Faber KJ, Ciarelli M, et al. Pull-out strength and stiffness of meniscal repair using absorbable arrows or Ti-Cron vertical and horizontal loop sutures. Am J Sports Med 1999;27: 626–31.

[95] Ghazavi MT, Pritzker KP, Davis AM, et al. Fresh osteochondral allografts for post-traumatic osteochondral defects of the knee. J Bone Joint Surg [Br] 1997;79(6):1008–13.

[96] Lobenhoffer P, Agneskirchner JD. Improvements in surgical technique of valgus high tibial osteotomy. Knee Surg Sports Traumatol Arthrosc 2003;11(3): 132–8.

[97] Gugenheim Jr JJ, Brinker MR. Bone realignment with use of temporary external fixation for distal femoral valgus and varus deformities. J Bone Joint Surg Am 2003;85-A(7):1229–37.

[98] Papageorgiou CD, Gil JE, Kanamori A, et al. The biomechanical interdependence between the anterior cruciate ligament replacement graft and the medial meniscus. Am J Sports Med 2001;29(2): 226–31.

[99] Barrack RL, Bruckner JD, Kneisl J, et al. Outcome of nonoperatively treated complete tears of the anterior cruciate ligament in active young adults. Clin Orthop Relat Res 1990;Oct(259):192–9.

[100] Bonamo JJ, Fay C, Firestone T. The conservative treatment of the anterior cruciate deficient knee. Am J Sports Med 1990;18(6):618–23.

[101] Cole BJ, Carter TR, Rodeo SA. Allograft meniscal transplantation: background, techniques, and results. Instr Course Lect 2003;52:383–96.

[102] Yoldas EA, Sekiya JK, Irrgang JJ, et al. Arthroscopically assisted meniscal allograft transplantation with and without combined anterior cruciate ligament reconstruction. Knee Surg Sports Traumatol Arthrosc 2003;11(3):173–82.

[103] Noyes FR, Barber-Westin SD. Irradiated meniscal allografts in the human knee: a two-to-five year follow-up study. Orthop Trans 1995;19:417.

[104] Rath E, Richmond JC, Yassir W, et al. Meniscal allograft transplantation. Two- to eight-year results. Am J Sports Med 2001;29(4):410–4.

[105] Shelton WR, Dukes AD. Meniscus replacement with bone anchors: a surgical technique. Arthroscopy 1994;10(3):324–7.

[106] Rodeo SA. Meniscal allografts–where do we stand? Am J Sports Med 2001;29(2):246–61.

[107] Rodeo SA, Seneviratne A, Suzuki K, et al. Histological analysis of human meniscal allografts. A preliminary report. J Bone Joint Surg Am 2000;82: 1071–82.

[108] Sekiya JK, Giffin JR, Irrgang JJ, et al. Clinical outcomes after combined meniscal allograft transplantation and anterior cruciate ligament reconstruction. Am J Sports Med 2003;31(6):896–906.

[109] Cole BJ, Rodeo S, Carter T. Allograft meniscus transplantation: indications, techniques, and results. J Bone Joint Surg Am 2002;84A:1236–50.

[110] Garrett JC, Stevenson RN. Meniscal transplantation in the human knee: a preliminary report. Arthroscopy 1991;7:57.

[111] Farley TE, Howell SM, Love KF, et al. Meniscal tear: MR and arthrographic findings after arthroscopic repair. Radiology 1991;180:517–22.

[112] Patten RM, Rolfe BA. MRI of meniscal allografts. J Comput Assist Tomogr 1995;19:243–6.

[113] Potter HG, Rodeo SA, Wickiewicz TL, et al. MR imaging of meniscal allografts: correlation with clinical and arthroscopic outcomes. Radiology 1996; 198:509–14.

[114] Verdonk R. Alternative treatments for meniscal injuries. J Bone Joint Surg Br 1997;79:866–73.

[115] Rijk PC, de Rooy TP, Coerkamp EG, et al. Radiographic evaluation of the knee joint after meniscal allograft transplantation. An experimental study in rabbits. Knee Surg Sports Traumatol Arthrosc 2002; 10(4):241–6.

ORTHOPEDIC
CLINICS
OF NORTH AMERICA

Orthop Clin N Am 36 (2005) 485 – 495

Biologic Approaches to Articular Cartilage Surgery: Future Trends

Nicholas A. Sgaglione, MD

North Shore University Hospital, Department of Orthopaedics, 600 Northern Boulevard, Great Neck, NY 11021, USA

The treatment of focal articular cartilage patho-logic conditions in the knee has become an area of great interest to clinicians, researchers, patients, and the media. Active, aging individuals who have symp-tomatic osteochondral defects will most certainly represent a considerable treatment challenge as the middle-aged population expands, cardiovascular and neoplastic disease treatments improve, and more em-phasis is placed on fitness and sport participation. The first of the baby boom generation will reach the age of 65 years in 2011. Increasing numbers of symptomatic chondral pathologic conditions will more than likely continue to present as patient demand for painless joint function is greater [1–4]. Furthermore, biologic repair methods for resurfacing articular cartilage defects of the knee continue to rapidly gain attention as more procedures become available and accepted as mainstream techniques [5]. Currently practitioners are able to arthroscopically stimulate a fibrous and fibrocartilagenous tissue heal-ing response through precise subchondral bone perfo-rations using marrow stimulation and microfracture techniques [6]. Viable transplantation of autologous osteochondral plugs using minimally invasive meth-ods is a reality, as is resurfacing of larger defects using cryopreserved and/or fresh allograft osteo-chondral tissue [7,8]. Successful ex vivo autologous chondrocyte culturing, expansion, and reimplantation have been clinically validated by reports of regener-ation of durable hyaline-like tissue at the site of complex articular cartilage defects that have been treated with autologous chondrocyte implantation (ACI) [9].

Despite these current approaches, the biologic treatment of hyaline cartilage disease in the knee remains controversial, unpredictable, and imprecise as far as indications are concerned, and is at times impractical as it relates to rehabilitation regimens and cost-effective delivery and recovery. Thus, challenges remain. Evidenced-based outcomes are limited, and although numerous techniques have been studied, few have been compared using controlled clinical trials. Presently, no one currently available method stands out as optimal, and many investigators con-tinue to favor multiple methods depending on clinical profiles related to patient age and activity levels, chondral pathoetiology, lesion site and size, and con-comitant pathology. Nonetheless, despite these limi-tations, what was once seemingly untreatable has now become the subject of enormous attention in the form of basic science projects, novel technologies, surgical techniques, and outcome investigations [10,11]. What is evolving is a multidisciplinary ap-proach to articular disease and osteoarthritis that brings together orthopedic clinicians, including total joint replacement surgeons, sports medicine specialists, and arthroscopists, and researchers and investigators in the fields of molecular biology, biochemistry, tissue engineering, and polymer sci-ence [12].

For the most part, many of the current surgical procedures may be considered first-generation meth-ods. As technology and knowledge progresses, the treatment approach to focal chondral pathology will improve. The expanding technologies and novel biologic treatment solutions for articular cartilage pathology hold great promise and most likely re-present only a fraction of what may be seen in the future [13–19]. Advances in noninvasive diagnostic

E-mail address: nas@optonline.net

0030-5898/05/$ – see front matter © 2005 Elsevier Inc. All rights reserved.
doi:10.1016/j.ocl.2005.05.006

imaging along with improvements in enhancing a more predictable and viable tissue repair or regeneration response are imminent realities [20–24]. This article reviews the current concepts of the biologic approach to articular cartilage pathology and discusses the future trends in the biologic approach to treatment of symptomatic articular cartilage focal defects.

Current approaches

There are various surgical procedures for treating symptomatic focal articular cartilage defects in the knee. All of these methods may play a role in the approach to chondral pathology, depending on lesion characteristics, clinical indications, patient profile and outcome goals, and surgeon preference and experience [25]. Chondral injury that does not penetrate the underlying subchondral bone has been shown to be associated with an unpredictable or absent healing response, whereas those defects that involve violation of the subchondral bone may result in a fibrous tissue healing scar repair response characterized by proliferation of type I collagen [26–28]. Stimulation and perforation of the subchondral base of focal chondral or osteochondral lesions remain the basis of marrow stimulation methods. Marrow stimulation techniques, including microfracture, can be performed arthroscopically and primarily at the point of an index arthroscopic surgical intervention to access the underlying vascular bone and release blood and associated marrow cells, resulting in pooling of an adhesive "superclot" at the site of the defect that then differentiates into a fibrous repair tissue [29]. The method of using arthroscopic awls to perforate the subchondral bony base of a chondral defect can be technically easy to perform with little associated morbidity. Longer-term reports of clinical success have been reported in more than 80% of patients treated with microfracture in an 11-year follow-up study [6]. A recently published, controlled-comparison, 2-year follow-up study yielded 75% clinical success, with evidence of hyaline-like tissue or fibrocartilage repair in 83% of cases that were examined histologically at follow-up in a prospective cohort of patients treated with microfracture (compared with those treated with autologous chondrocyte implantation) [30]. The limitation of marrow stimulation methods such as microfracture is the tendency for the treatment to unpredictably result in a fibrous or fibrocartilagenous tissue that may not respond in a durable and efficient manner to joint forces and

repetitive loading over time (at least compared with type II hyaline cartilage) [31]. In addition, although recent literature has compared the results of microfracture to autologous chondrocyte implantation, no controlled comparison studies have discussed the treatment of focal chondral defects with marrow stimulation versus debridement alone. The unpredictable natural history and course of chondral abnormalities are cited by one recent retrospective study of untreated chondral defects associated with anterior cruciate ligament tears, which found that at intermediate-term follow-up, many patients had not become symptomatic [32].

Osteochondral autograft transplantation has been described as an optimal method for transferring fully zoned native hyaline tissue, including the underlying bone tissue from an area of the knee that may see less-significant loading, to the pathologic site in the knee such as the trochlea and weight-bearing femoral condyles that are significantly loaded and the site and source of a symptomatic osteochondral lesion. This technique can be performed arthroscopically or using arthroscopically assisted methods and at the point of an index intervention, and has been shown to result in transfer of viable hyaline tissue that is securely press-fit [7,33]. Autograft transfer of osteochondral plugs theoretically provides a predictable source of zoned hyaline-like tissue using a less-invasive method with a shorter-term healing site profile. Several studies have reported good results in 79% to 92% of patients (depending on treated defect site) at intermediate-term follow-up [7,34–36]. The actual technique, however, can be challenging; in particular, restoring the precise surface anatomy of the condylar bevel or crown and the saddle-like curvature of the femoral trochlea [37–40]. Recent published reports indicate that technical issues such as graft size and harvest and press-fit insertion methods may clearly contribute to less than optimal results in certain cases [41,42]. Problems with perimeter integration, surface fibrillation, cleft formation, gapping, and cyst formation may be greater than originally appreciated. In addition, certain larger lesions can be difficult to treat and gain access to and the procedure is essentially limited by the number of grafts that can be harvested and the potential of harvest-site morbidity. One recent basic science report described the potential problem of perimeter chondrocyte death and tissue necrosis associated with harvesting osteochondral plugs [43–45].

Osteochondral allograft transplantation would seem to represent an optimal method for transplanting hyaline tissue, especially in the case where more extensive lesions are treated using larger allografts without any associated harvest site issues. At least in the salvage setting, the results of osteochondral allograft have been encouraging, with success reported in survivorship analysis in 95% of cases at 5 years postsurgery, 71% at 10 years, and 66% at 20 years [8,46–48]. Despite this success, the procedures are mostly performed using an arthrotomy rather than arthroscopically, and limitations in donor tissue availability and cost, disease transmission issues, and chondrocyte and tissue viability, particularly beyond 14 days, remain a concern [49–51].

ACI, which represents the first commercially approved biologic regenerative technology based on ex vivo chondrocyte culturing and staged reimplantation, has resulted in hyaline-like tissue with durable clinical and biomechanical results noted in 84% of cases with survivorship at extended follow-up [5,9, 52,53]. However, a more recent study found that at the 2-year follow-up of patients treated with ACI who underwent follow-up second-look tissue biopsies, only 39% of the treated defects were filled with hyaline cartilage, whereas 43% were filled with fibrocartilage and 18% with no healing tissue response at all. These histologic results were similar to a controlled comparison treatment study group that underwent microfracture, and both patient cohorts (at least at early 2-year follow-up) also had similar clinical outcomes [30]. ACI presently requires a two-staged procedure, the second of which includes an arthrotomy and the use of a periosteal patch to seal the cell-implanted lesion site. Periosteal harvesting and suturing is associated with more invasive surgery and has resulted in postoperative morbidity related to hypertrophy that may require subsequent surgical debridement [30]. These technical issues, in addition to stringent indications, cost concerns, and reimbursement controversies, have limited the widespread acceptance of this procedure.

Many of the currently available surgical options for chondral resurfacing have advantages and disadvantages. All of these treatment options have their proponents and detractors depending on clinical profiles, surgeon preference, primary and secondary approaches, and response to intervention. These treatment options can and may be associated with narrow or ill-defined indications and there is no one technique that stands out as an optimal surgical method that predictably restores zoned hyaline cartilage using a single-staged, minimally invasive method that is cost-effective and applicable to most of the significantly sized lesions indicated for surgery. The questions remain then: Can we do better? Can we improve on current methods? Can we obtain a more predictable repair tissue or better organized scar tissue using marrow stimulation? Can we limit the harvest issues

and potential morbidity associated with osteochondral transplantation, perhaps by using "off-the-shelf" site-specific allograft plugs? Can we improve the procurement, selection, and quality controlled processing and viability of allograft tissue? Can we improve the ex vivo expansion of chondrocytes to yield a more predictable cell line? Can we achieve a more robust and uniform hyaline tissue using next generation techniques that rely on three-dimensional scaffolds and arthroscopic delivery, obviating the need for injection of liquid suspensions of chondrocytes into sutured friable periosteal graft patches? Perhaps we can, but at what price and when? The task at hand is not easily reached within the context of emerging trends, such as cost-cutting, rushed rehabilitation, and biologic regulatory restraints. The goals, however, must remain high despite the difficulty of compiling controlled comparison data sets, rush to market by industry, and tendency for patients and physicians to impatiently grasp for the illusion of the "Holy Grail."

Clinical strategies

More recently, several trends have been observed in orthopedics and medicine in general that appear to be driving the introduction and development of newer treatment methods and technologies. There is a trend toward increasing emphasis on biologic approaches and solutions in orthopedics. Prosthetic arthroplasty has enjoyed considerable success over the last 35 years, yet limitations exist and the perfect artificial joint has not been found. Novel materials, polyethylene processing, and advances in trabecular metals continue to be introduced in an effort to improve prosthetic resurfacing durability. The issue of durability and survivorship has been heightened by the significant increase in the volume of joint replacement surgery considered and performed, especially in the 45- to 55-year-old age group of patients. This trend toward earlier arthroplasty has been fueled by the increasing popularity (and "reinvention") of unicompartmental arthroplasty. Concerns about durability and wear in this middle-aged patient population, and the inevitable need for revision with its attendant morbidity related to materials breakdown and associated bone loss, continue to remain a problem. These limitations and "burned bridges" will be of greater concern as patient life expectancies continue to increase and activity levels remain high. Biologic treatment options represent a viable solution for active middle-aged patients, as evidenced by the greater interest in corrective osteotomy surgery and viscosupplementation.

Another clear trend is the increased emphasis on minimally invasive procedures, which has captured the imagination of patients through direct-to-consumer advertising by medical device companies. In addition, as patients seek minimally invasive alternatives and essentially less pain compared with traditional procedures, many routinely expect faster healing, quicker recoveries, and accelerated rehabilitation. These expectations may be based on the small incisions, which do not necessarily impact the biologic remodeling and maturation that is associated with chondral resurfacing. These demands may then shape perceptions that can be magnified by the media, patients, and physicians, leading to unrealistic expectations regarding the manipulation of healing and biology.

Yet another trend is the increasing concern for cost-effective techniques that has become a significant reality as government and third-party insurers ratchet down on health care spending, cap certain procedures, and seek to define clinical treatment guidelines. Furthermore, orthopedic surgeons have increasingly entered into the ownership and management of surgery centers and have thereby rapidly become more aware and sensitive to the rising health care delivery costs and procedure-specific expenses.

Lastly, more precise MRI has increased the recognition and emphasis of articular cartilage pathologic conditions. Plain radiographs may not always reveal the true extent of chondral pathology, and arthroscopic evaluation frequently substantiates this diagnostic discrepancy. There are now increasing improvements underway in the area of noninvasive MRI of articular cartilage to better aid in the diagnosis of articular cartilage pathologic conditions. Specific MR techniques have been discussed, including high-resolution moderate TE fast spin-echo, three-dimensional fat-suppressed spoiled gradient-echo sequencing, delayed gadolinium-enhanced MRI of cartilage, and T2 collagen mapping [20,21,23,24]. More accurate and precise noninvasive diagnostic imaging methods specific to articular cartilage pathology, tissue repair response, and clinically correlative validation of symptoms, outcomes, and lesion resurfacing will serve to not only improve the ability to preemptively recognize abnormalities but also validate treatment regimens providing information about postsurgical tissue, type, percent fill, perimeter integration, and response to loading over time [22]. These trends pertaining to advances in biologic solutions, demand for minimally invasive procedures, and accelerated recovery, cost containment, and precise

noninvasive imaging may continue to drive or at least impact future clinical strategies and consideration of articular cartilage treatments.

Goals of treatment

The treatment goals of articular cartilage defects in the knee would include replacement, regeneration, or repair methods that result in hyaline tissue that integrates with native host tissue and functions durably under load and over time, and most importantly provides an asymptomatic joint [54]. The procedure to achieve this outcome would preferably be performed arthroscopically or using minimally invasive methods and be applicable at an index point of service intervention to ensure a single-staged surgery that is reasonably cost-effective and associated with minimal morbidity. Articular cartilage restoration requires re-establishing zoned hyaline cartilage that incorporates specifically arranged chondrocytes distributed in an extracellular matrix of fibrillar type II collagen with an adjacent transitional calcified zone and tidemark intimately interdigitated with the subchondral bone. The resurfacing of symptomatic articular defects more often (and particularly in cases of osteochondritis dissecans [OCD]) requires treatment and re-establishment of the subchondral bone. Multiple extrinsic and intrinsic factors may affect the technical approaches and clinical indications. Extrinsic factors include patient activity levels; functional demands placed on the knee; body mass index; lower extremity mechanical alignment and associated degenerative joint disease processes; ligament patholaxity; and meniscal attrition. Intrinsic factors include the site (eg, condyle location, trochlea, patella), size, perimeter (ie, geometric characteristics of the shoulders of the lesion), and depth of the defect and the complex interaction of biochemical and catabolic enzymatic processes that include cytokines and matrix metalloproteinases. The more precise approach to articular cartilage defects in the future will most likely require consideration of patient and site-specific treatments to address some of these factors, and more precise control of catabolic processes in addition to anabolic enhancement [11,19,25].

Controversy remains over how clinical outcomes are determined. Outcome success is presumably measured by the elimination and absence of pretreatment symptoms such as site-specific pain, effusion, and catching. Over what period of time is that success measured? Does success actually mean elimination of symptoms, or that progression to osteoarthritis will be halted or just limited over a certain time frame? Are we defining a "bridge" procedure that buys time and temporizes the ultimate solution of joint arthroplasty? Is clinical success good enough or do we demand specific tissue fill, and to what extent and with what type of tissue? Should we not also use mechanical measures to evaluate the repair tissue response to load? Are microindentation probes that quantitate the stiffness of the repair tissue compared with healthy native host hyaline cartilage a truer measure of success? Is tissue fill with hyaline cartilage assessed and measured arthroscopically or using newer non-invasive MRI technologies? Is the extent of tissue fill always clinically correlative with a durable response to loading and presumed symptom resolution? These questions for the most part remain unanswered and need to be defined as more surgical techniques are introduced.

Future approaches

Currently available treatments, marrow stimulation, or microfracture promote tissue repair, whereas ACI could be considered a first-generation regeneration technique, and osteochondral transplantation may be considered biologic replacement. Whether repair, regeneration, or replacement techniques are selected, there are several key components that would be essential to optimize the production of new articular cartilage tissue. One component would be a chondroprogenitor cell source for replication, biologic turnover, and most importantly extracellular matrix production. The methodology used for targeting the chondroprogenitor cell line may vary and can include treatments that directly affect the native cells and tissue (eg, using an exogenous bioactive polypeptide injected or applied to the lesion intra-articularly). Another method may include transplantation of the actual chondroprogenitors onto a scaffold from an exogenous but autogenous source or from a separate allogeneic site. The cell line may also be treated in an ex vivo manner to activate the cells to produce a more robust extracellular matrix. Finally, an actual expanded and fully formed tissue may be transplanted after potential exogenous ex vivo treatments either with bioactive factors or extrinsic biomechanical or biophysical stimulation (eg, using a bioreactor in which in vitro cyclic compressive stimulation is applied to expanded tissue cultures to induce a more exuberant cellular response and extracellular matrix product). The requirements for successful hyaline tissue production as far as chondroprogenitor lines

are concerned would include cellular proliferation, differentiation, phenotypic expansion, perimeter and deep integration, and tissue maturation. A selected cell line would be expanded to proliferate and phenotypically express chondrocytic functions to produce extracellular matrix and proteoglycan macro-molecules that more expeditiously impart optimal biomechanical function [55–57].

Sources of chondroprogenitor cell lines include mesenchymal stem cells, immature or juvenile chondrocytes, and differentiated chondrocytes (as used in ACI). Several sources of stem cells exist, including those from bone marrow elements and muscle, dermal, adipose, and periosteal tissue. Furthermore, autogenous versus allogeneic cell lines may be selected depending on availability, cost-effectiveness, and compatibility. The advantages of using autogenous cell lines and tissue include reduced cost and negligible disease transmission and immunologic issues, whereas the advantages of allogeneic sources include availability and reduced harvest site issues and morbidity [58,59].

A second essential component that would be required for regeneration of new tissue would be a porous scaffold to act as a delivery vehicle for the selected chondroprogenitors and to provide a unique three-dimensional structure within the site of a focal defect that is to be treated. A matrix or scaffold would provide surface structure to facilitate cell migration, attachment, and stability, and afford porosity or void volume to allow cell expansion, angiogenesis (where applicable), and tissue maturation to proceed in a stable manner [60,61]. The immature composite tissue would initially require an organizational architecture and temporary load sharing during the potentially lengthy proliferative and maturation phases of repair and regeneration. The tissue construct, including the scaffold, would require a method of attachment to the underlying bone tissue and adjacent native articular cartilage. Numerous scaffolds have been discussed and continue to evolve as novel biomaterials and polymers are developed. Scaffolds may be purely biologic in nature (collagen, hyaluronate, alginate, submucosal xenograft, dermal allografts), whereas others are mineral-based (tricalcium phosphate, hydroxyapatite, calcium sulfate) and still others are carbohydrate-based (polylactide, polyglycolide, polycaprolactone) [60–64]. Recently, the author used novel bilayered mineral-based/polylactide/polyglycolide-based and fiber-reinforced composite polymer and calcium sulfate bone graft substitute plugs for resurfacing intra-articular OCD bony defects and osteochondral fractures in the knee [19]. Preliminary study has been initiated demon-

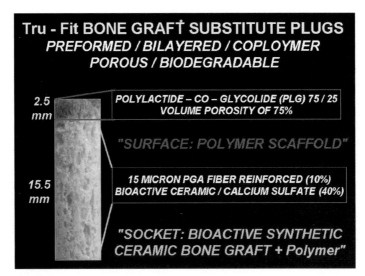

Fig. 1. 9 × 18-mm-long (5-, 7-, 9-, and 11-mm diameters) intra-articular bilayered (polylactide–glycolide surface/polymer–fiber reinforced calcium sulfate base) bone graft substitute. (*Courtesy of* OsteoBiologics, San Antonio, TX; with permission.)

strating clinical safety and efficacy (OsteoBiologics, San Antonio, Texas) (Figs. 1–3).

A third key component of advancing new tissue regeneration would include the use of bioactive factors that may be used to amplify cell expansion, strengthen phenotype, improve extracellular matrix production, and at the same time reduce cell breakdown and catabolic degradation. These complex proteins can be classified according to their actions as anabolic agents or morphogens and growth factors that function to amplify chondrocyte phenotype and differentiation, improve the quality of the matrix expression, and thereby produce a purer and more optimal and durable hyaline tissue. Several proprietary preparations of bioactive bone morphogenic

proteins (BMP-2 and BMP-7) were recently released for clinical use in the treatment of bony nonunion and fusion procedures. Other bioactive proteins that can be classified as catabolic inhibitors act to control and limit degradative processes, tissue breakdown, and cell death or apoptosis. Bioactive polypeptides can have numerous functions and may act on adjacent host tissue as mitogens and chemotactic agents that permit manipulation and control of biologic processes, including healing, repair, and regeneration [64–67]. Actual delivery of bioactive growth factors currently remains an issue. Questions remain regarding whether they should be introduced directly at the

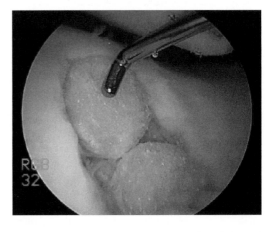

Fig. 3. Arthroscopic view of resurfaced lateral femoral condyle chondral defect with copolymer resorbable bone graft substitute scaffolds.

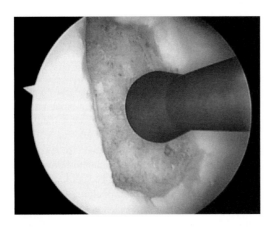

Fig. 2. Osteochondral fracture of lateral femoral condyle.

site of treatment in vivo or indirectly using ex vivo methodologies, or whether they should be impregnated within a scaffold and be carrier-based. The use of gene-modified cell-based therapies may hold the answer, as chondroprogenitor cell lines may be modified in the laboratory using candidate genes that encode for selected morphogenic proteins that enhance healing. Those tissue-engineered cell lines can then be delivered to the treatment site to amplify and promote healing and regeneration [68–71]. Despite much promising preclinical work, clinical applications are still limited by control, dosing, half-life, safety, and cost issues. This technology awaits more definitive bioassays for documentation of specific growth factor presence, concentration, stability, expression, and effective action, and more substantial evidenced-based clinical validation [72].

The recent reports of platelet-rich plasma (PRP) have stimulated much interest in the potential for a "one-stop," intraoperative, cost-effective, practical method for introducing and capturing "growth factors" within an operating room setting. The use of concentrated autogenous PRP theoretically loaded with growth factors may play a role in the treatment of a drilled chondral defect to amplify the superclot that forms. The use of ready-to-mix concentrates of the patient's own blood products prepared at the time of the surgical procedure may represent the first example of the introduction of the clinically practical application of bioactive factors to the surgical site. In addition, centrifuged and intraoperatively prepared PRP may be used with biocompatible scaffolds to "seed" the acellular constructs and perhaps achieve a more predictable fibrous repair tissue. The requirements for successful tissue repair methodology would then include cells, scaffold, and bioactive factors, with each part of the approach balanced and titrated to ultimately produce viable repair tissue (Fig. 4).

Next-generation cell-based therapies

A new generation of cell-based therapies has been introduced in Europe, implanting ex vivo–expanded autogenous chondrocytes onto novel collagen and hyaluronic acid (HA)–based scaffolds. These methods would eliminate the use of periosteal patch grafts. There is also the increased potential for arthroscopic application that would theoretically reduce the invasiveness and morbidities associated with current ACI methods. Several resorbable scaffolds have been used, including extracellular xenograft collagen membranes and esterified nonwoven HA matrices that function as the cell-seeded platforms for ex vivo impregnation of the autogenous chondrocytes. These

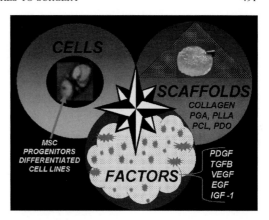

Fig. 4. Cell source, scaffold matrix, and bioactive growth factor schematic for tissue repair. EGF, epidermal growth factor; IGF-1, insulinlike growth factor; MSC, mesenchymal stem cells; PCL, polycaprolactone; PDGF, platelet-derived growth factor; PDO, polydiaxanone; PGA, polyglycolic acid; PLLA, polylactic acid; TGFB, transforming growth factor β; VEGF, vascular endothelial growth factor.

membrane or matrix-associated autologous chondrocyte implantations (MACI) methods and HA-based scaffolds (Hyalograft C/Hyaff 11, Fidia Advanced Biopolymers, Albano Terme, Italy) provide the potential to implant a three-dimensional chondrocyte-seeded construct that can be either press-fit into the chondral defect or attached using minimally invasive suturing techniques, bioadhesives, or bioabsorbable anchors. They clearly have several advantages over first-generation ACI techniques, but although initial clinical data appear encouraging, the Food and Drug Administration has not yet approved these methods for clinical use in the United States (see Fig. 4) [61,63].

Another novel cell-based technology that has successfully completed preclinical testing in a porcine animal model in this country is based on a technique that uses autologous chondrocytes that are seeded onto a bovine collagen sponge (NeoCart, Histogenics, Malden, Massachusetts). The three-dimensional construct is then statically cultured ex vivo and expanded, and then placed in a computerized cyclic hydrostatic loading chamber using a nutrient-rich perfusate and controlled low oxygen and gas environment. Exposure to biophysical stimuli using external bioreactor technology has been shown to promote better-defined chondrogenic phenotype and robust extracellular matrix with greater potential for successful hyaline tissue expansion and perimeter integration. On completion of the 6-week laboratory treatment, the mature construct is then implanted into the chondral defect using a miniarthrotomy or potentially arthroscopic technique and held in place using a proprietary bioadhesive. This methodology is currently undergoing a phase 1 clinical study (A. Kusanagi, PhD, personal communication, 2004).

Efforts to enhance chondrocytic phenotype expression during ex vivo cell culture expansion have begun to receive attention. Clinical trials have been initiated in Europe using proprietary methods to precisely select optimal chondrogenic phenotypes to study the potential benefits of using chondrocyte cell markers. This phenotypic profiling may have value in achieving a more robust hyaline tissue regeneration in explant culture expansions, thereby optimizing future ACI methods [56,57].

Gene-modified tissue engineering

The enormous potential that gene-modified therapy and tissue engineering hold has generated significant interest in all of medicine and particularly in orthopedics. The ability to manipulate articular cartilage tissue repair or generate tissue is an exciting concept. Gene therapy may be defined as the ability through gene transfer to deliver a therapeutic protein to a target cell or tissue to induce that cell or tissue to engage in repair or regeneration and guide healing [13–15,18,69,71,72].

Gene-modified tissue engineering involves the selection of a candidate gene that specifically codes for expression of a therapeutic protein that then contributes to articular cartilage repair or regeneration. The gene would then be introduced into a selected target cell line, such as a chondrocyte or stem cell, that would be then manufacture and express the therapeutic protein. Introduction of the candidate gene and encoding DNA into the selected target cell could be performed using viral transfection or non-viral methods and using ex vivo or in vivo techniques. Once the gene has transduced the target cell, it would then function as a source of the therapeutic protein or bioactive factors that on release would presumably result in a higher-quality structural repair tissue. Mechanisms to control the process would need to be programmed into the sequence using genes for promoters; cell line purification and phenotype expression; timing and dosing of the protein production; and shutting it down ("suicide genes").

Recent projects have centered on the introduction of genes coding for chondrogenic morphogens, including insulinlike growth factor, platelet-derived growth factor, basic fibroblast growth factor, and transforming growth factor beta (TGF-β), including the bone morphogenetic proteins (BMP-2, BMP-4, and BMP-7) [66]. BMP-7 and IGF-1 have been shown to improve the quality of the expressed chondral tissue through stimulation of proteoglycan synthesis and proliferation of chondrocytes, whereas the sonic hedgehog (Shh) protein is part of a family of polypeptide regulators that function "upstream" of the traditional chondrocyte-regulating growth factors (TGF-β). Initial experiments have been directed toward repairing chondral defects using these gene-modified approaches, and encouraging laboratory results have been observed. The resultant hyaline cartilage constructs have been noted to have superior characteristics compared with untreated controls [73].

We are not there yet

Despite the rapid developments that continue to be directed toward providing a solution for treating articular cartilage pathology, many limitations still exist. The expansion and application of laboratory and bench-top results to the clinical setting remain incomplete. There continues to be difficulty applying projects that have realized success in the smaller-animal model to a viable larger-animal experimental model that more optimally replicates human clinical trials. There have been problems obtaining site-specific zonal hyaline tissue that predictably integrates with the subchondral bone and surrounding normal native tissues. Bioactive factor applications remain elusive and in some respect are still a clinical "leap of faith." Their safety, dosing, control, and cost-effectiveness remain unclear. The use of gene-modified protocol, stem cells, and bioactive factors is still in its infancy. Tremendous hurdles remain as we face increasingly stringent government regulatory issues, politically charged legalities, and media-driven public safety concerns. Most importantly, there continues to be a need for cost-effective interventions that are equally practical and acceptable to clinicians and patients.

Summary

There is much promise on the horizon as we continue to expand efforts to find a more successful treatment approach to symptomatic focal articular cartilage lesions in the knee. Advances in basic science and clinical progress will continue to propel an increased emphasis on biologic approaches to surgical resurfacing and restoration. Current methods have come a long way in a short period of time, yet there is more to go. This is, however, an exciting time in which molecular biologists, bioengineers, polymer chemists, and clinical orthopedists are all at work to find solutions. The future holds much promise, and although many rapid advances have been made and progress has been realized, much work still needs to done. Many questions need to be answered and many problems solved before a reproducible and more predictable methodology can be realized. Connective tissue progenitor cell lines, allogeneic tissue, novel biocompatible scaffolds, and bioactive factors will all play a role as work in these areas expands. Our targets must remain realistic and our goals practical, yet the quest for valid data analysis, evidenced-based controlled clinical studies, and interpretations must be encouraged. We are certainly moving in the right direction as far as the future of biologic cartilage restoration is concerned, but we are not there yet.

References

[1] Williams R, Wickiewicz T, Warren R. Management of unicompartmental arthritis in the anterior cruciate deficient knee. Am J Sports Med 2002;8:749–60.

[2] Aroen A, Loken S, Heir S, et al. Articular cartilage lesions in 993 consecutive knee arthroscopies. Am J Sports Med 2004;32:211–5.

[3] Hjelle K, Solheim E, Strand T. Articular cartilage defects in 1,000 knee arthroscopies. Arthroscopy 2002; 18:730–4.

[4] Curl W, Krome J, Gorgon ES. Cartilage injuries: a review of 31,516 knee arthroscopies. Arthroscopy 1997; 13:456–60.

[5] Sgaglione N, Miniaci A, Gillogly S, et al. Update on advanced surgical techniques in the treatment of traumatic focal articular cartilage lesions of the knee. Arthroscopy 2002;18:9–32.

[6] Steadman JR, Briggs K, Rodrigo J, et al. Outcomes of microfracture for traumatic chondral defects of the knee: average 11-year follow-up. Arthroscopy 2003; 19:477–84.

[7] Hangody L, Fules P. Autologous osteochondral mosaicplasty for the treatment of full thickness defects of weight-bearing joints; ten years of experimental and clinical experience. J Bone Joint Surg Am 2003; 85(Suppl 2):25–32.

[8] Gross A. Fresh osteochondral allografts for post-traumatic knee defects: surgical technique. Op Tech Orthop 1997;7(4):334–9.

[9] Peterson L, Brittberg M, Kiviranta I, et al. Autologous chondrocyte transplantation; biomechanics and long-term durability. Am J Sports Med 2002;30:2–12.

[10] Alford J, Cole B. Cartilage restoration, part 1 basic science, historical perspective, patient evaluation, and treatment options. Am J Sports Med 2005;33:295–306.

[11] Alford J, Cole B. Cartilage restoration, part 2 techniques, outcomes, and future directions. Am J Sports Med 2005;33:443–60.

[12] Buckwalter JA. Integration of science into orthopaedic practice: implications for solving the problem of articular cartilage repair. J Bone Joint Surg Am 2003; 85(Suppl 2):1–7.

[13] Bruder S. Current and emerging technologies in orthopaedic tissue engineering. Clin Orthop 1999; 376(Suppl):S406–9.

[14] Hannallah D, Peterson B, Lieberman J, et al. Gene therapy in orthopaedic surgery. J Bone Joint Surg Am 2002;84(6):1046–61.

[15] Jackson D, Simon T. Tissue engineering principles in orthopaedic surgery. Clin Orthop 1999;367S:S31–45.

[16] Jackson DW, Scheer MJ, Simon TM. Cartilage substitutes: overview of basic science and treatment options. J Am Acad Ortho Surg 2001;9:37–52.

[17] Musgrave D, Fu F, Huard J. Gene therapy and tissue engineering in orthopaedic surgery. J Am Acad Orthop Surg 2002;10(1):6–15.

[18] Sgaglione N. The biological treatment of focal articular cartilage lesions in the knee: future trends? Arthroscopy 2003;19:154–60.

[19] Sgaglione N. The future of cartilage restoration. J Knee Surg 2004;17:235–43.

[20] Burstein D, Gray M. New MRI techniques for imaging cartilage. J Bone Joint Surg Am 2003;85(Suppl. 2): 70–7.

[21] Burstein D, Gray M. Potential of molecular imaging of cartilage. Sports Med Arthros Rev 2003;11(3):182–91.

[22] Brown W, Potter H, Marx R. Magnetic resonance imaging appearance of cartilage repair in the knee. Clin Orthop 2004;422:214–23.

[23] Hooper T, Potter H. Imaging of chondral defects. Op Tech Orthop 2001;11:76–82.

[24] Potter H, Linklater J, Allen A. Magnetic resonance imaging of articular cartilage in the knee: an evaluation with use of fast-spin-echo imaging. J Bone Surg Am 1998;80:1276–84.

[25] Sgaglione N. Decision-making and approach to articular cartilage surgery. Sports Med Arthros Rev 2003;11: 192–201.

[26] Guilak F, Fermor B, Keefe F, et al. The role of biomechanics and inflammation in cartilage injury and repair. Clin Orthop 2004;423:17–26.

[27] Menche D, Frenkel S, Blair B, et al. A comparison of abrasion burr arthroplasty and subchondral drilling in the treatment of full-thickness cartilage lesions in the rabbit. Arthroscopy 1996;12:280–6.

[28] O'Driscoll S. The healing and regeneration of articular cartilage. J Bone Joint Surg Am 1998;80(12): 1795–807.

[29] Frisbie D, Oxford J, Southwood L, et al. Early events in cartilage repair after subchondral bone microfracture. Clin Orthop 2003;407:215–27.

[30] Knutsen G, Engbretsen L, Ludvigsen T. Autologous chondrocyte implantation compared with microfracture in the knee: a randomized trial. J Bone Joint Surg Am 2004;86:455–64.

[31] Nehrer S, Spector M, Minas T. Histologic analysis of tissue after failed cartilage repair procedures. Clin Orthop 1999;365:149–62.

[32] Shelbourne KD, Jari S, Gray T. Outcome of untreated traumatic articular cartilage defects of the knee. J Bone Joint Surg Am 2003;85(Suppl 2):8–16.

[33] Barber A, Chow J. Arthroscopic osteochondral transplantation: histologic results. Arthroscopy 2001;17: 832–5.

[34] Chow JC, Hantes M, Houle JB. Arthroscopic autogenous osteochondral transplantation for treating knee cartilage defects: a 2 to 5 year follow-up study. Arthroscopy 2004;20:681–90.

[35] Hangody L, Fules P. Autologous osteochondral mosaicplasty for the treatment of full – thickness defects of weight-bearing joints. J Bone Joint Surg Am 2003;85:25–32.

[36] Horas U, Pelinkovic D, Aigner T. Autologous chondrocyte implantation and osteochondral cylinder transplantation in cartilage repair of the knee joint: a prospective comparative trial. J Bone Joint Surg Am 2003;85(2):185–92.

[37] Koh J, Wirsing K, Lautenschlager E, et al. The effect of graft height mismatch on contact pressures following osteochondral grafting. Am J Sports Med 2004; 32:317–20.

[38] Terukina M, Fujioka H, Yoshiya S, et al. Analysis of the thickness and curvature of articular cartilage of the femoral condyle. Arthroscopy 2003;19:969–73.

[39] Pearce S, Hurtig M, Clarnette R, et al. An investigation of 2 techniques for optimizing joint surface congruency using multiple cylindrical osteochondral autografts. Arthroscopy 2001;17:50–5.

[40] Bartz R, Kamaric E, Noble P, et al. Topographic matching of selected donor and recipient sites for osteochondral autografting of the articular surface of the femoral condyles. Am J Sports Med 2001;29: 207–12.

[41] Evans P, Miniaci A, Hurtig M. Manual punch versus power harvesting of osteochondral grafts. Arthroscopy 2004;20:306–10.

[42] Duchow J, Hess T, Kohn D. Primary stability of pressfit–implanted osteochondral grafts. Am J Sports Med 2000;28:24–7.

[43] Huntley J, Bush P, McBurnie J. Chondrocyte death associated with human femoral osteochondral harvest as performed for mosaicplasty. J Bone Joint Surg Am 2005;87:351–60.

[44] Garretson R, Katolik L, Beck P, et al. Contact Pressure at osteochondral donor sites in the patellofemoral joint. Am J Sports Med 2004;32:967–74.

[45] Simonian P, Sussman P, Wickiewicz T, et al. Contact pressures at osteochondral donor sites in the knee. Am J Sports Med 1998;26(4):491–4.

[46] Shasha N, Krywulak S, Backstein D, et al. Long term follow-up of fresh tibial osteochondral allografts for failed tibial plateau fractures. J Bone Joint Surg Am 2003;85(Suppl 2):33–9.

[47] Chu CR, Convery FR, Akeson WH, et al. Articular cartilage transplantation: clinical results in the knee. Clin Orthop 1999;360:159–68.

[48] Convery RF, Akeson WH, Meyers MH. The operative technique of fresh osteochondral allografting of the knee. Op Tech Ortho 1997;7:340–4.

[49] Williams R, Drees J, Chen C. Chondrocyte survival and material properties of hypothermically stored cartilage. An evaluation of tissue used for osteochondral allograft transplantation. Am J Sports Med 2004; 32(1):132–9.

[50] Williams S, Amiel D, Ball S, et al. Prolonged storage effects on the articular cartilage of fresh human osteochondral allografts. J Bone Joint Surg Am 2003; 85(11):2111–20.

[51] Vangsness T, Garcia I, Mills CR, et al. Allograft transplantation in the knee: tissue regulation, procurement, processing and sterilization. Am J Sports Med 2003;31:474–81.

[52] Peterson L, Minas T, Brittberg M, et al. Treatment of osteochondritis dissecans of the knee with autologous chondrocyte transplantation. J Bone Joint Surg Am 2003;85(Suppl 2):17–24.

[53] Minas T, Peterson L. Advanced techniques in autologous chondrocyte transplantation. Clin Sports Med 1999;18(1):13–44.

[54] Poole R. What type of cartilage repair are we attempting to attain? J Bone Joint Surg Am 2003; 85(Suppl 2):40–4.

[55] Benya P, Shaffer J. Dedifferentiated chondrocytes reexpress the differentiated collagen phenotype when cultured in agarose gels. Cell 1982;30:215–24.

[56] De Bari C, Dell'Accio F, Luyten F. Human periosteum-derived cells maintain phenotypic stability and chondrogenic potential throughout expansion regardless of donor age. Arthritis Rheum 2001;44:85–95.

[57] Dell'Accio F, De Bari C, Luyten F. Molecular markers predictive of the capacity of expanded human articular chondrocytes to form stable cartilage in vivo. Arthritis Rheum 2001;44:1608–19.

[58] Diduch D, Jordan L, Mierisch C, et al. Marrow stromal cells embedded in alginate for repair of osteochondral defects. Arthroscopy 2000;16(6):571–7.

[59] Schreiber R, Ilten-Kirby B, Dunkelman N, et al. Repair of osteochondral defects with allogeneic tissue engineered cartilage implants. Clin Orthop 1999;367S: 382–95.

[60] Grande D, Halberstadt C, Naughton G, et al. Evaluation of matrix scaffolds for tissue engineering of articular cartilage grafts. J Biomed Mater Res 1997;34: 211–20.

[61] Cherubino P, Ronga M, Grassi F, et al. Autologous chondrocyte implantation with a collagen membrane. J Orthop Surg (Hong Kong) 2002;1:169–77.

[62] Nettles D, Vail TP, Morgan M, et al. Photocrosslinkable hyaluron as a scaffold for articular cartilage repair. Ann Biomed Eng 2004;32:391–7.

[63] Warren S, Sylvester K, Chen C, et al. New directions in bioabsorbable technology. Orthopedics 2002;25(10): 1201–10.

[64] Hickey D, Frenkel S, Di Cesare P. Clinical applications of growth factors for articular cartilage repair. Am J Orthop 2003;2:70–6.

[65] Sellars R, Zhang R, Glasson S, et al. Repair of articular cartilage defects one year after treatment with recombinant human bone morphogenetic protein-2 (rhBMP-2). J Bone Joint Surg Am 1997;79(10):1452–63.

[66] Mason J, Grande D, Barcia M, et al. Expression of human bone morphogenic protein 7 in primary rabbit periosteal cells: potential utility in gene therapy for osteochondral repair. Gene Ther 1998;5:1098–104.

[67] Cook S, Patron L, Salkeld S, et al. Repair of articular cartilage defects with osteogenic protein-1 (BMP-7) in dogs. J Bone Joint Surg Am 2003;85(Suppl 3): 116–23.

[68] Fortier L, Balkman C, Sandell L, et al. Insulin-like growth factor-I gene expression patterns during spontaneous repair of acute articular cartilage injury. J Orthop Res 2000;19:720–8.

[69] Grande D, Mason J, Dines D. Stem cells as platforms for delivery of genes to enhance cartilage repair. J Bone Joint Surg Am 2003;85(Suppl 2):111–6.

[70] Mason J, Brietbart A, Barcia M, et al. Cartilage and bone regeneration using gene-enhanced tissue engineering. Clin Orthop 2000;379(Suppl):S171–8.

[71] Muschler G, Nakamoto C, Griffith L. Engineering principles of clinical cell based tissue engineering. J Bone Joint Surg Am 2004;86:1541–8.

[72] Grande D, Breidbart A, Mason J, et al. Cartilage Tissue engineering: current limitations and solutions. Clin Orthop 1999;367S:S176–85.

[73] Riddle R, Johnson R, Laufer E, et al. Sonic hedgehog mediates the polarizing activity of the ZPA. Cell 1993;75:1401–16.

ORTHOPEDIC
CLINICS
OF NORTH AMERICA

Orthop Clin N Am 36 (2005) 497–504

High Tibial Osteotomy for the Treatment of Unicompartmental Arthritis of the Knee

Annunziato Amendola, MD*, Ludovico Panarella, MD

Department of Orthopaedics, University of Iowa Hospitals and Clinics, 200 Hawkins Drive, 01018 JPP, Iowa City, IA 52242-1088, USA

High tibial osteotomy has to be considered a valuable option in the surgical management of knee osteoarthritis. Localized wear in the knee corresponds to a malalignment that is either causative of or contributory to the arthritis. For many years, the value of osteotomy to correct malalignment has followed the principle of transferring load to the unaffected compartment of the knee to relieve symptoms and slow disease progression, and has been used extensively, with techniques becoming more refined over time [1]. In addition, despite good long-term results with total knee arthroplasty, there remains a significant concern regarding the longevity of these prostheses, particularly in younger patients. In contrast, osteotomy provides an alternative that preserves the knee joint and, when appropriately performed, should not compromise later arthroplasty if it becomes necessary. The reported results of high tibial osteotomy vary considerably across the literature, but the procedure generally provides good relief of pain and restoration of function in approximately 80% to 90% of patients at 5 years, and 50% to 65% at 10 years [2–7]. In the analysis of these results, most authors have found that success is directly related to achieving optimal alignment [3,6,8]. Accurate preoperative assessment and technical precision are therefore essential to achieving satisfactory outcomes. Many techniques have been described for proximal tibial osteotomies. This article discusses the various options available for alignment correction in the treatment of osteoarthritis

using proximal tibial osteotomy and outlines the appropriate indications and technique.

Patient selection

A patient is typically a candidate for high tibial osteotomy when the orthopedic surgeon can clinically detect a varus standing alignment associated with (1) medial compartment arthrosis in a stable knee (classical indication); (2) medial compartment arthrosis with associated ligament deficiency and instability (such as anterior cruciate ligament [ACL], posterior cruciate ligament, posterolateral corner, or combined ligament deficiencies); or (3) painful medial knee compartment with associated medial meniscus deficiency, articular cartilage defects requiring resurfacing, or osteochondritis dissecans lesions.

These conditions often require high tibial osteotomy to unload the affected compartment in either a combined or staged procedure.

Indications in the unicompartmental osteoarthritis of the older active patient

High tibial osteotomy is appropriated for young, active patients who have primary degenerative arthritis involving a single compartment in a malaligned limb. Patient selection is more difficult with older patients. In the United States, osteotomies have substantially decreased in the past 2 decades [9]. Over the age of 60 years, knee replacements are typically offered. Considering the success of arthroplasty in

* Corresponding author.
E-mail address: ned-amendola@uiowa.edu
(A. Amendola).

this age group, osteotomy is frequently proposed as an alternative to joint replacement [10]. The motivation of the patient is crucial. Patients who have high physical demand are usually willing to find a solution that will not dramatically decrease the activity level. Nevertheless, the patient should be aware that the pain relief may not be complete and everlasting. At physical examination, patients should have a complete range of motion, a stable knee, and asymptomatic lateral and patellofemoral compartments. Contraindications that may be considered relative for a younger patient become absolute in older patients,. The authors believe that high tibial osteotomy is still a valuable option in medial unicompartmental arthritis in a strongly motivated older patient when osteoarthritis is associated with a varus deformity of the knee.

Preoperative assessment

Clinical assessment

To achieve success with proximal tibial osteotomy, the selection of the appropriate patient is crucial. A thorough clinical assessment requires a detailed history and physical examination followed by appropriate imaging. Specific analysis of this information will help determine whether or not a patient is likely to benefit from osteotomy. Important aspects of a patient's general history include age, occupation, activity level, and medical and surgical history. Particularly significant are the patient's expectations of postoperative activity. Questions specific to the knee include previous injury and surgery, and effectiveness of previous treatment. The patient may have noticed an increasing deformity or a static long-term malalignment. Pain history should focus on the site, severity, and aggravating and relieving factors. History of locking, catching, or instability may point to a mechanical source of symptoms, and the specific details of each of these symptoms should be sought to determine if other procedures, such as arthroscopy, may be beneficial as an adjunct to osteotomy.

Physical examination should commence with an overall impression of the patient's health and build. Lower limb alignment should be assessed at each level and the gait should be observed for any abnormalities, particularly a thrust in the direction of the deformity, indicating a significant dynamic component. Presence of deformity in all of three planes should be assessed, particularly rotational deformity

because this is more difficult to assess later radiographically. Whether or not a deformity is fixed or correctable should be determined. Patellar tracking and the presence of crepitus are noted. Presence of an effusion is assessed and location of tenderness should be recorded carefully. Range of motion is measured, particularly looking for the presence of a flexion contracture and the amount of flexion comfortably achieved. Ligaments are examined, including sagittal plane laxity and the presence of coronal plane pseudo-laxity, indicating loss of effective joint space. Reproduction of clicking symptoms and pain with McMurray's test may indicate a meniscal tear. Grinding of medial and lateral compartments through the midflexion range may reproduce symptoms from the diseased compartment, and also roughly mimic the effect of an osteotomy by loading the unaffected compartment. Adjacent joints are examined, and assessment of neurovascular function is essential.

Radiographic assessment

Knee radiographs are an essential component of preoperative assessment. The standard assessment at the authors' institution includes four short films and one full leg alignment film. The four short films are bilateral anteroposterior weight-bearing radiographs taken at full extension, bilateral posteroanterior weight-bearing radiographs at 45° of flexion, and lateral and skyline films of the affected leg. Full-length alignment films can be single-leg standing, double-leg standing, or supine, and the various advantages of each have been cited by several investigators [11,12]. Whichever is used, it is critical to be aware of the implications of each view. Supine views may underestimate the correction required for the weight-bearing situation, and single-leg films may overestimate correction because of the component of soft tissue laxity not requiring a bony correction. Unfortunately, at this stage there is not a general agreement on the most accurate method of radiographic assessment. It is the authors' practice to obtain single-leg standing films from hips to ankles and to assess the joint congruency angle as an indication of the component of deformity because of soft tissue laxity. The lateral laxity can then be taken into account when calculating the desired correction [11]. Several measurements are taken from these films to help with preoperative planning. Most important are the axis of weight-bearing, the joint-congruency angle, and the individual articular angles of tibia and femur to assess the site of the deformity. The axis of weight-bearing is a straight line drawn from the center of the hip to the center of the ankle, showing where the weight passes through the knee joint. Mechanical and anatomic axes of the knee are also measured. The congruency angle between tibial and femoral articular surfaces is recorded, and the angle between these surfaces and the axes of the respective shafts gives an indication of degree of deformity in tibia and femur. Lateral radiographs are assessed for sagittal plane deformity, including measurement of tibial slope.

Calculations of corrections

Several methods have been described for measuring the required correction on preoperative radiographs [11,13,14]. The general principle is to determine the desired postoperative location of the weight-bearing line and thereby calculate the angular correction necessary to achieve this.

Principles of varus knee correction

The varus knee with medial compartment osteoarthritis is certainly the most common scenario for which osteotomy has been used. As Coventry [13] advocated, the results of high tibial osteotomy in this scenario have been best when the anatomical axis is corrected to 8° to 10° of valgus [3]. However, too much overcorrection may yield poor results, particularly in ligamentously lax individuals, in whom minimal bony overcorrection may lead to a significant clinical deformity. Other researchers have examined this in relation to the site of the weight-bearing line, with best results seen when this passes through the lateral plateau at 62% to 66% of the width of the plateau [11]. Preoperative assessment has therefore aimed to achieve this outcome. The traditional method is to measure the preoperative mechanical and anatomic axes and calculate the angular correction necessary to produce 2° to 4° of mechanical or 8° to 10° of anatomic valgus. Dugdale and colleagues [11] and Miniaci and colleagues [14] described more recent methods. These methods determine the angular correction necessary to place the postoperative weight-bearing line at 62% to 66% of the width of the tibial plateau. The current technique used at the authors' institution is that of Dugdale and colleagues [11], calculating the correction to 62.5% of the tibial plateau width, which equates to 3° to 5° of mechanical valgus. Excess deformity from soft tissue laxity is accounted for by subtracting the increase in congruency angle when compared with the unaffected leg on the double-leg

standing film, or a non–weight-bearing film of the affected leg. By measuring the width of the tibia at the level of the proposed osteotomy, the surgeon can convert the angular correction into a wedge size, particularly for opening wedge osteotomies.

Surgical techniques

Medial opening wedge osteotomy

Medial opening wedge osteotomy has not been as widely reported in the English-speaking literature as the closing wedge technique, but has been extensively used in Europe and is now enjoying increased popularity in North America [15,16]. The theoretical advantages of opening wedge over closing wedge include (1) restoration of anatomy with addition of bone to the diseased medial side; (2) the ability to achieve predictable correction in coronal and sagittal planes; (3) the ability to adjust correction intraoperatively; (4) the requirement for only one bone cut; (5) avoidance of proximal tibiofibular joint disruption and invasion of the lateral compartment; and (6) the relative ease of combining with other procedures such as ACL reconstruction.

The disadvantages of this procedure include the creation of a defect that requires bone graft with attendant harvest morbidity, a theoretical higher risk for nonunion, and a longer period of restricted weight-bearing postoperatively. Medial opening wedge osteotomy has been the preferred technique in the authors' institution for these reasons.

Graft choices include autograft, allograft, or pre-prepared bone substitutes. Each option has its own advantages and disadvantages, and although iliac crest autograft probably remains the current gold standard, it has recently been the authors' practice to use femoral head allograft. Using femoral head allograft avoids donor site morbidity and decreases surgical time. This method seems to result in predictable union, but it obviously requires a readily available bone bank facility.

The surgery is performed with the patient supine on the operating table. A radiolucent table is used with a leg extension applied to allow fluoroscopic visualization of hip, knee, and ankle joints for alignment assessment intraoperatively. A tourniquet is placed around the thigh and the involved limb is prepared and draped free. If iliac crest bone autograft is to be used, the ipsilateral crest is also prepared and draped. The surgeon stands with the instruments on the opposite side of the operating table to the operative leg, allowing direct access to the medial side of the leg. This positioning also allows the fluoroscopy arm to come in from the operative side.

A skin marker is used to identify the medial joint line, the tibial tubercle and patellar tendon, and the posteromedial border of the tibia. The leg is elevated and the pneumatic tourniquet inflated. A 5-cm longitudinal incision is created, extending from 1 cm below the medial joint line midway between the medial border of the tubercle and the posteromedial border of the tibia. The sartorius fascia is exposed by sharp dissection. The superior border of the sartorius fascia is identified, and the pes is then retracted distally with a blunt retractor, exposing the superficial fibers of the medial collateral ligament. The anterior border of the medial ligament is identified and this is raised with a scalpel and periosteal elevator. A blunt Hohmann retractor is then passed deep to the medial ligament, around the posteromedial corner of the proximal tibia, and along the posterior cortex of the tibia to protect the posterior neurovascular structures. The medial border of the patellar tendon is next identified. A short longitudinal incision is made to allow a second blunt lever to be placed deep to the patellar tendon just proximal to the tubercle and retract it laterally. The medial insertion of the tendon is released for a few millimeters to allow clear identification of the anterosuperior corner of the tubercle. The residual retinaculum and periosteum between these anterior and posterior retractors is then elevated toward the joint line, creating a proximally based flap. Elevation of this flap gives a subperiosteal exposure of the tibia from the tibial tubercle around to its posteromedial corner. A guidewire is then inserted along the line of the proposed osteotomy. Accurate positioning of this guidewire is critical to the success of the operation. The two points of the superomedial corner of the tibial tubercle and the tip of the head of the fibula laterally are identified. The guidewire starting point on the anteromedial tibia is the direct continuation of a straight line between these two points, which usually gives a start point on the medial tibia approximately 3 to 4 cm distal to the medial joint line. Guidewire obliquity can be altered somewhat depending on the size of the tibia and the required size of correction (a more oblique osteotomy will allow for only a small angle of correction). Fixation failure and intra-articular fracture are more likely with increased obliquity of the osteotomy [17]. The guidewire should be placed about 2 mm proximal and parallel to the proposed osteotomy, because the osteotomy is performed on the distal side of the guidewire. The obligatory requirements for wire position include osteotomy placed above the

patellar tendon insertion; medial start position distal enough to allow sufficient bone for positioning of the fixation plate on the proximal fragment; osteotomy at least 1 cm distal to the tibial articular surface at its most proximal (lateral) extent; and osteotomy directed toward the upper end of the proximal tibiofibular articulation. The tibial osteotomy is performed immediately distal to the guide pin, the pin protecting against proximal migration of the osteotomy into the joint. The slope of the osteotomy in the sagittal plane is critical and should mimic the proximal tibial joint slope. The tendency to make the osteotomy perpendicular to the long axis of the tibia should be avoided because this will create a thin bony fragment posteriorly because of the natural posterior tibial slope of approximately $10°$. The joint line can be palpated through the incision or marked with needles, and the line of the osteotomy should be equidistant from the medial joint line anteriorly and posteriorly to be parallel to the tibial slope. The authors mark the tibia along this line with a cautery device before performing the osteotomy. With the previously placed retractors protecting the soft tissues anteriorly and posteriorly, a small oscillating saw is used to cut the tibial cortex from the tibial tubercle around to the posteromedial corner under direct vision. Thin, flexible osteotomes are then used to advance the osteotomy laterally, systematically working from medial to lateral and anterior to posterior. The osteotomy should be taken to within 1 cm of the lateral tibial cortex, using intermittent fluoroscopy. As much as possible should be completed with the thin osteotomes, and this is completed using solid, broad but thin osteotomes. In the authors' early experience with this technique, intra-articular fractures were caused by using thicker, traditional osteotomes. A useful technique to ensure completeness of the osteotomy is to place a broad osteotome centrally to open the osteotomy slightly, and then work with a long, thin osteotome along the anterior and posterior cortices. While performing the osteotomy, it is important to regularly check progress with a fluoroscope to ensure the appropriate depth and direction of the cut. Calibrated guide pins and osteotomes are also available and can help keep the requirement for fluoroscopy to a minimum. The mobility of the osteotomy is checked by gentle manipulation of the leg with a valgus force. Ensure the osteotomy opens slightly before proceeding with the wedge osteotome. If the osteotomy seems incomplete, check again with a narrow flexible osteotome anteriorly and posteriorly. "Stacking osteotomes" can often be useful in encouraging mobility in the osteotomy. The Puddu tapered osteotome is then engaged into the osteotomy, keeping the direction parallel to the osteotomy. This osteotome is calibrated to allow assessment of the size of the opening achieved in millimeters, and should be advanced slowly (roughly 5 mm/min) to allow gradual opening of the osteotomy. Fluoroscopy should be used to ensure progression of the instrument parallel to the osteotomy. Rapid advancement is likely to produce unwanted extension of the osteotomy proximally or laterally. Alignment should be checked intermittently. Once the calculated preoperative wedge size has been reached, a long alignment rod can be used as described earlier with fluoroscopy. With the rod centered over the hip and ankle joints, it should lie at 62% to 66% of the tibial width, usually at the lateral edge of the lateral tibial spine. The sagittal plane correction should also be assessed by looking carefully at the amount of opening of the osteotomy anteriorly and posteriorly. Because the tibia is a triangular bone-in cross-section with apex anterior, the size of the wedge anteriorly at the tubercle should be less than that at the posteromedial corner to avoid changing the tibial slope. If the gap is anteriorly equal to that at the posteromedial corner, the posterior slope of the tibia will be inadvertently increased. The sagittal alignment is also important, and the orientation of the tibial articular surface in this plane is another critical determinant of outcome. In cases of pure medial compartment osteoarthritis in a stable knee, the normal tibial slope should be preserved using the method described previously and intraoperative fluoroscopy. The sagittal slope can be deliberately altered in instability patterns to decrease tibial translations and assist with knee stability [18]. A decreased posterior tibial slope will decrease anterior tibial translation in the presence of ACL deficiency. This decrease may be important to address in medial compartment arthritis subsequent to chronic ACL deficiency, and in anterior instability patterns with associated varus deformity. Conversely, in the posterior cruciate–deficient knee, increasing the tibial slope can be beneficial by increasing anterior tibial translation.

The slope can be adjusted by the type of plate used and its positioning. Plates are available in symmetrical rectangular or tapered shapes. Positioning a symmetrical plate anteromedially will increase the slope; using a tapered plate directly medially should have no effect on slope; and positioning a tapered plate posteromedially should decrease tibial slope. Once the desired correction has been achieved and plate positioning determined, the insertion handle from the Puddu osteotome is removed, leaving the tines in situ. The plate is placed between these tines,

which can then be removed. The plate is fixed with two partially threaded 6.5-mm cancellous screws proximally and two 4.5-mm fully threaded screws distally. Fluoroscopic guidance should be used for the proximal screws to avoid penetration into either the joint or the osteotomy. The defect is then grafted using the preferred bone graft as discussed earlier. It has been the authors' practice in defects of 7.5 mm or less to use only cancellous chips, and in defects of 10 mm or greater to use cancellous chips in the lateral aspect of the defect and two corticocancellous wedges medially: one anterior and one posterior to the plate. Final fluoroscopic assessment ensures adequate position of the osteotomy and hardware and complete filling of the defect with bone graft. The wound is irrigated and a suction drain placed against bone posteromedially. Closure is completed in layers and dry dressing applied to the wounds.

A standard postoperative regimen is followed that is somewhat more restricted than that for the closing wedge procedure. For the first 6 weeks, the knee is placed in a range of motion brace set at 0° to 90°, and the patient is encouraged to achieve this range, particularly full extension. During this period, the patient remains touch weight-bearing using crutches. From week 6 to 12 the brace is discontinued and weight-bearing is progressed gradually to full weight-bearing over the 6-week period. From 3 to 6 months postoperatively, the patient is encouraged to progress activities as tolerated. Short radiographs are taken at 6 and 12 weeks to ensure maintenance of position and healing, and long-leg alignment films are performed at 6 months to assess the correction achieved.

Lateral closing wedge osteotomy

The most commonly reported osteotomy for medial compartment osteoarthritis is the lateral closing wedge osteotomy, popularized by Coventry [1] and Insall and colleagues [19]. The goal is correction of alignment as outlined earlier, achieved by removing a laterally based wedge of bone and closing the resultant defect. Many variations of technique have been described for this procedure [1,2, 11,19], with the general principle the same in all. Traditionally, an angular calculation is converted to a wedge size based on the tibial width, although newer instrument systems provide angled cutting jigs, obviating this conversion. It is important when calculating a wedge size not to use the traditional rule of 1° equating to 1 mm, because this will lead to an undercorrection in virtually every tibia.

Knee arthroscopy may be required before beginning the osteotomy to treat mechanical symptoms.

This procedure is performed on the basis of a pre-operative assessment, suggesting an intra-articular source of mechanical symptoms. The authors do not routinely perform arthroscopy to assess the lateral and patellofemoral compartments, or if symptoms such as pain and swelling are attributable to the arthritis rather than arthroscopically treatable pathologic conditions such as unstable meniscal tears or loose bodies.

The authors use the L-shaped skin incision, with the vertical limb along the lateral edge of the tibial tubercle and the horizontal limb parallel and 1 cm distal to the lateral joint line, taken posteriorly to the anterior aspect of the fibular head. Dissection is performed to expose the fascia of the anterior compartment, which is incised along the anterolateral crest of the tibia, leaving a 5-mm cuff for later closure. A Cobb elevator is used to elevate the muscle from the anterolateral surface of the tibia, and the iliotibial tract is elevated from Gerdy's tubercle proximally, inserting a stay suture for retraction and later closure. The common peroneal nerve is not routinely exposed but is palpated and protected throughout the procedure. Treatment of the proximal tibiofibular joint also has many described techniques, including joint excision or disruption, fibular osteotomy, or excision of the fibular head. The authors prefer to disrupt the joint but preserve the fibular head. The proximal tibiofibular joint is exposed, the anterior capsule incised, and a curved osteotome is directed posteromedially to disrupt this articulation and mobilize the fibula so as not to impede later correction. A Z-shaped retractor is placed through this joint along the posterior aspect of the tibia to protect posterior soft tissues. It is critical that this retractor be placed directly against bone along the posterior cortex to protect the neurovascular structures [20,21]. The lateral edge of the patellar tendon is identified, and a second Z retractor placed underneath it to protect it during the osteotomy. In this way, the proximal tibia is exposed from tibial tubercle to the posterolateral cortex and is therefore prepared for the osteotomy. In removing a laterally based wedge, either an angular cutting guide can be used or a specific-size wedge can be removed. The authors' preferred technique is to remove the outer cortex and large portion of the wedge with saw cuts, then remove the medial half using a combination of curettes, rongeurs, and osteotomes before closing the osteotomy. Otherwise, there is a significant risk for intra-articular fracture. In performing these cuts, it is important to check the position of anterior and posterior retractors to ensure soft tissue protection and to cut the anterior and posterior cortices

fully, to within 1 cm of the medial cortex. The fluoroscope can be used to assist with assessment of completeness of wedge removal. Once closed, position and alignment are checked with the fluoroscope and fixation then completed. Fixation is usually completed with two stepped staples or alternatively an Association for the Study of Internal Fixation (ASIF) L- or T-shaped plate. Wound closure is then completed as described earlier. A drain is placed against bone and closure is completed in layers. Fascial closure is interrupted and should attempt to cover the plate as much as is possible without undue tension.

Postoperative management involves use of a hinged brace for 6 weeks, with partial weight-bearing using crutches during this time. Radiographs are taken at the 6-week mark, and if early healing of the osteotomy is evident, the brace is discontinued and the patient progressed to weight-bearing as tolerated. A second radiograph is performed at the 3-month mark. If the osteotomy is united, activity level can be increased as tolerated. A long-leg alignment film is taken at the 6-month mark to assess the accuracy of the correction.

Dome osteotomy

The dome osteotomy was originally popularized by Maquet [22] and has been advocated by some authors for correction of large deformities [22–24]. The main advantage of this procedure is that it allows essentially unrestricted correction in contrast to the more commonly used techniques. The position of the tibial tubercle in relation to the joint line is unaffected, and Maquet actually advocated anterior displacement of the tubercle through the osteotomy. Use of an external fixator allows postoperative adjustment of alignment, which may be an advantage especially in larger corrections, although the risk for possible pin tract infection and the cumbersome nature of the treatment for patients is a potential disadvantage.

Achieving a gradual correction with an external fixator

Use of an external fixator to achieve a gradual correction has several potential advantages over a single-stage correction, with many authors reporting good results with this technique [16,25–27]. First, large corrections may be technically impossible with standard closing or opening wedge techniques, either because of excessive bone removal compromising fixation and creating deformity in the closed wedge technique or excessive soft tissue tension in the opening wedge technique. External fixators also allow constant manipulation of the alignment during the healing process to optimize alignment [16]. This constant manipulation is an especially attractive feature for larger deformities in which major bony deformity combined with soft tissue laxity can make prediction of a single-stage correction difficult. Circular external fixators also allow easy manipulation of angular and translational correction in all three planes as necessary [25].

These advantages are balanced by the significant drawbacks of possible pin site infection [26–28], which if not successfully treated can lead to deeper infection and compromise later surgery, particularly arthroplasty. The treatment is also a significant ordeal for the patient, who needs to be compliant with treatment and prepared for alterations in lifestyle during the treatment period. Selection of the most appropriate patient for this technique is probably the most important factor in the success of the procedure.

It has recently been the authors' practice to use a circular hybrid external fixator for the correction of deformities that are technically beyond the standard medial opening wedge procedure. In addition, in these larger deformities it is not possible to accurately predict the appropriate single-stage correction. The specific device the authors use is a hybrid ring fixator that has six obliquely oriented struts initially set to match the patient's deformity, and then gradually adjusted to bring the rings parallel. Computer software (Taylor Spatial Frame; Smith and Nephew, Memphis, Tennessee) allows input of deformity parameters from preoperative radiographs and subsequently calculates initial strut settings and a correction rate set by the surgeon based on specific soft tissue structures at risk. These calculations allow preoperative construction of the frame. It is essential to schedule a preoperative appointment with the patient to show and size the frame and to explain the procedure and postoperative schedule. Ring circumference should allow for two fingerbreadths of clearance from soft tissue circumferentially.

The construct the authors use is a single ring attached to the proximal fragment and two parallel rings attached to the distal fragment, which provides a stable construct.

The procedure is performed with the patient supine on a radiolucent table. A computer in the operating room allows adjustments in the parameters that may prove necessary during the course of frame application. A tourniquet is not necessary, and the leg is draped free. Bolsters are placed under the thigh and foot, allowing for circumferential access to the tibia from knee to ankle. The frame is sized and constructed preoperatively, and is checked once more to ensure appropriate fit on the patient's leg. A fine wire is passed from lateral to medial parallel to the joint surface, at least 10 mm distal to the joint to minimize the risk for intrasynovial penetration with possible infection. The frame is applied to this wire and, using the undersurface of the frame as a template, a second fine wire is passed, taking care to keep the frame parallel to the joint surface in coronal and sagittal planes. The frame is then secured distally using a fine wire across the distal ring. The construct is then completed by adding two 5-mm half-pins to each ring. It is important to use the subcutaneous surface of the tibia as much as possible and avoid penetration of anterior compartment musculature. The proximal ring fixation should be at the level of or proximal to the tibial tubercle.

The osteotomy is then performed percutaneously at the lower border of the tibial tubercle through two small incisions using a Gigli saw subperiosteally. The two anterior struts are disconnected from the middle ring and deflected to facilitate performing the osteotomy. Wounds are closed and pin sites dressed, and the osteotomy is left static for 10 days, after which the correction is then performed gradually by the patient at home, usually over a 7- to 14-day period, depending on the degree of deformity. Range of motion as tolerated is allowed immediately, and touch weight-bearing is performed for the first 10 days while pin site wounds heal. Thereafter, partial weight-bearing with crutches is allowed. At the end of the initial correction, a long standing weight-bearing film is taken, parameters are re-entered into the computer software, and any necessary residual correction can be performed until optimal alignment is achieved. The frame is removed after healing is confirmed radiologically and clinically.

Summary

Proximal tibial osteotomy can be used to correct varus and valgus deformities in the management of isolated medial or lateral compartment osteoarthritis.

Several surgical techniques have been described for achieving this goal, and the relative merits of each have been outlined. Whatever the technique used, the selection of the appropriate patient and the attainment of a precise correction without complications are critical to the success of the procedure. If these goals are met, proximal tibial osteotomy should provide long-term relief of pain and restoration of function in patients who have localized knee osteoarthritis even in carefully selected, highly motivated, older active patients.

References

[1] Coventry MB. Upper tibial osteotomy. Clin Orthop 1984;182:46–52.
[2] Billings A, Scott DF, Camargo MP, et al. High tibial osteotomy with a calibrated osteotomy guide, rigid internal fixation, and early motion: long-term follow-up. J Bone Joint Surg Am 2000;82:70–9.
[3] Coventry MB, Ilstrup DM, Wallrichs SL. Proximal tibial osteotomy: a critical long-term study of eighty-seven cases. J Bone Joint Surg Am 1993;75:196–201.
[4] Insall JN, Joseph DM, Msika C. High tibial osteotomy for varus gonarthrosis: a long-term follow-up study. J Bone Joint Surg Am 1984;66:1040–8.
[5] Ivarsson I, Myrnerts R, Gillquist J. High tibial osteotomy for medial osteoarthritis of the knee: a 5 to 7 and 11 year follow-up. J Bone Joint Surg Br 1990;72:238–44.
[6] Naudie D, Bourne RB, Rorabeck CH, et al. The Insall Award: survivorship of the high tibial valgus osteotomy: A 10- to 22-year followup study. Clin Orthop 1999;367:18–27.
[7] Rinonapoli E, Mancini GB, Corvaglia A, et al. Tibial osteotomy for varus gonarthrosis: a 10- to 21-year follow-up study. Clin Orthop 1998:185–93.
[8] Yasuda K, Majima T, Tsuchida T, et al. A ten- to 15-year follow-up observation of high tibial osteotomy in medial compartment osteoarthrosis. Clin Orthop 1992:186–95.
[9] Trousdale RT. Osteotomy: patient selection, preoperative planning, and results. In: Callaghan JJ, Rosenberg AG, Rubash HE, et al, editors. The adult knee. Philadelphia: Lippincott Williams & Wilkins; 2002. p. 985–90.
[10] Sprenger TR, Doerzbacher JF. Tibial osteotomy for the treatment of varus gonarthrosis. Survival and failure analysis to twenty-two years. J Bone Joint Surg Am 2003;85A(3):469–74 [Erratum in: J Bone Joint Surg Am 2003;85A(5):912.].
[11] Dugdale TW, Noyes FR, Styer D. Preoperative planning for high tibial osteotomy: the effect of lateral tibiofemoral separation and tibiofemoral length. Clin Orthop 1992:248–64.
[12] Ogata K, Yoshii I, Kawamura H, et al. Standing radiographs cannot determine the correction in high tibial osteotomy. J Bone Joint Surg Br 1991;73:927–31.
[13] Coventry MB. Upper tibial osteotomy for osteoarthritis. J Bone Joint Surg Am 1985;67:1136–40.

[14] Miniaci A, Ballmer FT, Ballmer PM, et al. Proximal tibial osteotomy: a new fixation device. Clin Orthop 1989:250–9.
[15] Hernigou P, Medevielle D, Debeyre J, et al. Proximal tibial osteotomy for osteoarthritis with varus deformity: a ten to thirteen-year follow-up study. J Bone Joint Surg Am 1987;69:332–54.
[16] Magyar G, Ahl TL, Vibe P, et al. Open-wedge osteotomy by hemicallotasis or the closed-wedge technique for osteoarthritis of the knee: a randomised study of 50 operations. J Bone Joint Surg Br 1999;81:444–8.
[17] Amendola A, Mrkonjic L, Clatworthy M, et al. Opening wedge high tibial osteotomy using a novel technique: early results and complications. J Knee Surg 2004;17:164–9.
[18] Amendola A, Giffin R, Sanders D, et al. Osteotomy for knee instability: the effect of increasing tibial slope on anterior tibial translation. Presented at Specialty Day of American Orthopaedic Society for Sports Medicine. San Francisco, CA. February 28–March 4, 2001.
[19] Insall J, Shoji H, Mayer V. High tibial osteotomy: a five-year evaluation. J Bone Joint Surg Am 1974;56:1397–405.
[20] Smith PN, Gelinas J, Kennedy K, et al. Popliteal vessels in knee surgery: a magnetic resonance imaging study. Clin Orthop 1999:158–64.
[21] Georgoulis AD, Makris CA, Papageorgiou CD, et al. Nerve and vessel injuries during high tibial osteotomy combined with distal fibular osteotomy: a clinically relevant anatomic study. Knee Surg Sports Traumatol Arthrosc 1999;7:15–9.
[22] Maquet P. Valgus osteotomy for osteoarthritis of the knee. Clin Orthop 1976;00:143–8.
[23] Takahashi T, Wada Y, Tanaka M, et al. Dome-shaped proximal tibial osteotomy using percutaneous drilling for osteoarthritis of the knee. Arch Orthop Trauma Surg 2000;120:32–7.
[24] Sundaram NA, Hallett JP, Sullivan MF. Dome osteotomy of the tibia for osteoarthritis of the knee. J Bone Joint Surg Br 1986;68:782–6.
[25] Catagni MA, Guerreschi F, Ahmad TS, et al. Treatment of genu varum in medial compartment osteoarthritis of the knee using the Ilizarov method. Orthop Clin North Am 1994;25:509–14.
[26] Klinger HM, Lorenz F, Harer T. Open wedge tibial osteotomy by hemicallotasis for medial compartment osteoarthritis. Arch Orthop Trauma Surg 2001;121:245–7.
[27] Weale AE, Lee AS, MacEachern AG. High tibial osteotomy using a dynamic axial external fixator. Clin Orthop 2001:154–67.
[28] Geiger F, Schneider U, Lukoschek M, et al. External fixation in proximal tibial osteotomy: A comparison of three methods. Int Orthop 1999;23:160–3.

ORTHOPEDIC
CLINICS
OF NORTH AMERICA

Orthop Clin N Am 36 (2005) 505–512

The UniSpacer: A Treatment Alternative for the Middle-aged Patient

Richard H. Hallock, MD

Orthopedic Institute Of Pennsylvania, 875 Poplar Church Road, Camp Hill, PA 17036, USA

The UniSpacer (Zimmer, Inc., Warsaw, IN) is a metallic tibial hemiarthroplasty for treatment of isolated osteoarthritis of the medial compartment of the joint. It is a mobile-bearing, self-centering shim that is introduced into the knee through a limited medial arthrotomy without requiring bone cuts or fixation to the tibia or femur. Clinical data are now available that define the efficacy of the procedure in addition to defining the ideal clinical setting for its use in the treatment of osteoarthritis of the medial compartment of the knee.

Osteoarthritis of the medial compartment of the knee leaves the medial compartment partially devoid of articular and meniscal cartilage. The collapse of the compartment shifts the weight-bearing of the knee into varus alignment. Two degrees of varus leads to 75% of the load shifted to the medial compartment. Two degrees of valgus leads to 50/50 load distribution between the compartments. Thus, just a 4° correction of alignment shifts 25% of the load off the medial compartment. Acting as an intra-articular shim, the results of radiograph review demonstrate that the UniSpacer corrects the axial alignment from an average of 2.2° of varus to an average of 2.7° of valgus, thus off-loading the medial compartment by more than 25%.

The UniSpacer does not require any bone resection for implantation and has no bone fixation. Bone and ligament preservation allows for future procedures to be performed without compromise. There is no currently available hemiarthroplasty that allows for the same degree of anatomic preservation of the knee as the UniSpacer. Eliminating fixation also

allows the device to be used in certain patients, especially the obese, without the fear that mechanical failure may result from stresses at the bone/cement/implant interface. Because the device is not fixed to the bone, failure from loosening or stress riser fracture is not possible. These two new design premises combined with the prior history of the McKeever/McIntosh [1–3] allow the UniSpacer to fill a niche as a "bridge" procedure for younger patients trying to preserve their anatomy for future, yet probably inevitable, total knee replacement (TKR)s. This rationale is similar to that used in the employment of a high tibial osteotomy, but without the potential morbidity or alteration of the tibial joint line.

Patient profile

At this time, the UniSpacer is only indicated for the treatment of osteoarthritis of the medial compartment of the knee. Implantation of the UniSpacer is a major surgical procedure and should be used on patients who have failed less invasive treatment options and still have significant pain and functional limitations. Most patients will have had treatment with nonsteroidal anti-inflammatory drugs, viscosupplementation, and arthroscopic techniques. The radiograph axial alignment is varus with loss of joint space (Fig. 1).

Indications/contraindications

As with any surgical procedure, the success of the operation depends significantly on patient selection.

E-mail address: rhhallock@aol.com

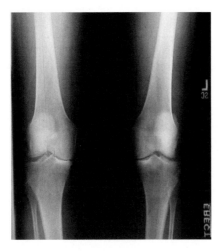

Fig. 1. Radiograph of varus knee with loss of joint space.

Proper selection is a multifactorial issue based on patient demographics; degree of pain and disability; physical parameters of the knee; radiographic analysis; and most importantly, patient expectations. As a bridge procedure, this device is ideally suited for the younger patient. The younger patient will not only be concerned with immediate pain relief, but also the condition of the knee over a 30- to 50-year period of treatment. Thus patients in the 35- to 55-year-old age category have most to gain from this device. Patients older than 65 years remain better candidates for conventional unicompartmental knee replacement (UKR) and TKR because pain relief still remains a higher priority than bone and ligament preservation. With all the subchondral bone preserved, obesity is not a contraindication. Because obesity is a relative contraindication for UKR and osteotomy, the UniSpacer does offer the obese patient an alternative not previously available. Similar to body weight, gender is neither an indication nor a contraindication. There may, however, be men and women who do not wish to have an osteotomy strictly on the basis of cosmesis. Some patients simply do not wish to have the necessary valgus realignment of their leg from the osteotomy, especially if their alignment is already valgus before their medial compartment degeneration.

This operation has two major benefits: knee preservation and pain relief. Preoperative pain intertwines directly with postoperative expectations. This procedure is an interpositional arthroplasty. Patients may expect that pain relief will be approximately 80% improvement over the preoperative level. Patients must be informed that pain relief will not be 100% in most cases. The pain relief will be predictably less complete than alternative low-friction arthroplas-

ties, and patients must be fully aware of this preoperatively to avoid unfair comparison to UKR or TKR postoperatively. Avoiding the pitfalls of selection for this procedure is difficult because of the high patient demand for any less invasive procedure in general. Any patient older than 65 years should routinely be considered for a traditional procedure such as TKR or UKR. The obvious advantage of knee preservation is lost on these older patients.

Patients require full extension postoperatively to obtain an optimal result. Any patient with a preoperative flexion contracture will have the same contracture postoperatively because the UniSpacer procedure does not release soft tissues. Without normal knee extension, the postoperative UniSpacer patient will not regain a normal gait pattern, which can produce a whole complex of lower extremity and lumbar spine complaints. Ligament stability is also critical for success. The anterior cruciate ligament (ACL) must be intact for stability of the implant. An ACL-deficient knee must be reconstructed or the patient should be deselected for this implant. The relative motion between the tibia and femur in the ACL-deficient knee creates too much shear force to allow comfortable, controlled translation and rotation of the implant between flexion and extension. The UniSpacer will follow the femoral condyle during flexion. This femoral roll back is exaggerated in the ACL-deficient knee. The UniSpacer will translate off the posterior aspect of the tibial plateau in an ACL-deficient knee during flexion (Figs. 2 and 3).

Finally, the UniSpacer is a low-demand prosthesis. As such, the patient should avoid impact activities

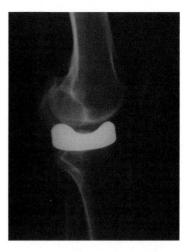

Fig. 2. Lateral radiograph of an ACL-deficient knee in extension with the UniSpacer positioned under the femoral condyle.

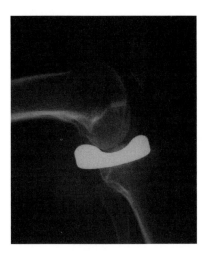

Fig. 3. Lateral radiograph of an ACL-deficient knee in flexion demonstrating exaggerated femoral rollback and posterior positioning of the UniSpacer.

after implantation. Although the implant will not fail with impact activity, the UniSpacer knee, which still has arthrosis, will develop pain and effusion after high-impact activities. A younger patient who has greater physical demands is still better served by a high tibial osteotomy (HTO).

Preoperative radiology

The patient should have a minimal amount of preoperative radiology. Four view radiographs, including anterior-posterior (AP) erect, lateral, tunnel, and skyline views, should be obtained. The degeneration seen on radiograph should be limited to the medial compartment of the joint. The AP-erect view must demonstrate joint space narrowing and varus axis deviation. If the cartilage space in the medial compartment is not narrowed, there will be no potential space to insert the device, and thus any space-occupying implant will essentially "overstuff" the medial compartment. On the other hand, advanced disease with severe medial compartment bone deformity is also a contraindication. Medial femoral subluxation is usually associated with bone loss on medial aspect of the medial tibial plateau. This bone loss creates a dome-shaped tibial plateau, which is also a contraindication. The lateral view radiograph is important in evaluating long-standing ligament instability. Anterior subluxation of the tibia implies chronic ACL deficiency, and posterior subluxation

of the tibia implies chronic posterior cruciate ligament (PCL) deficiency. ACL and PCL insufficiency are contraindications for UniSpacer surgery for the reasons described in the indications section. The radiograph in Fig. 4 demonstrates anterior translation of the tibia relative to the femur, indicating long-standing ACL insufficiency. The MRI is also a useful tool in evaluating the integrity of the ACL/PCL in cases where the history and clinical examination are questionable.

Osteophytes seen on the notch view suggest a severity of degeneration that may not be obvious on the AP and lateral views alone. Although not a direct contraindication, they should cause caution when indicating a patient. Patients who have notch osteophytes may not only have excessive degeneration of the medial or lateral compartments of the knee but they may also have degenerative tears of the ACL. The skyline view is important in evaluating patella femoral arthrosis. It is occasionally difficult to distinguish symptoms of medial disease from patellafemoral (PF) disease, so this view may confirm disease with the presence of osteophytes along the border of the PF joint, subluxation of the patella, or joint space narrowing especially in the lateral facet of the PF joint. The surgeon must clearly distinguish between medial compartment symptoms and patellofemoral symptoms to avoid the problem of patients who have significant unexpected postoperative patellofemoral pain. Clinical correlation of the radiology with patient history and physical examination is necessary to avoid the pitfalls of patient selection.

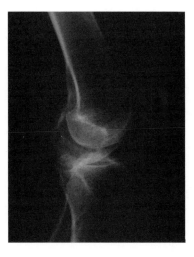

Fig. 4. Lateral radiograph of a chronic ACL-deficient knee with posterior positioning of the femoral condyle in relation to the tibia.

Surgical technique

The surgical technique for the UniSpacer initially begins with an arthroscopic evaluation of the joint. This evaluation allows the surgeon to fully assess the extent of degeneration in the patellofemoral joint, medial compartment, and lateral compartment of the knee. Mild chondrosis in the patellofemoral joint and lateral compartment are acceptable; however, anything more than grade II chondromalacic changes in either of these two areas remains a relative contraindication for implantation of the UniSpacer. The integrity of the ACL and the extent of degeneration in the medial compartment must also be assessed. If the ACL is not intact, the UniSpacer should not be implanted unless plans are made to reconstruct the ACL in the future. Any significant deformity to the subchondral bone plate of the tibial plateau is also a relative contraindication. Full thickness loss of articular cartilage on either the femoral condyle or the tibial plateau, however, does not preclude implantation of the device. Most candidates, in fact, will have bipolar full-thickness loss of articular cartilage. The medial compartment in a typical UniSpacer candidate is illustrated in Fig. 5.

Following the arthroscopic evaluation, a median parapatellar arthrotomy is made from the midpatella down to the tibial joint line (Fig. 6).

Then, a mobile window is created by undermining the subcutaneous tissue, and the medial retinaculum is incised from the superior pole of the patella down to the tibial joint line. The anteromedial structures are then elevated off of the upper 2 cm of the medial tibia only if there are significant osteophytes along the upper medial border of the tibia. Osteophytes are then resected using a rongeur along the medial femur from the femoral sulcus to the posterior aspect of the

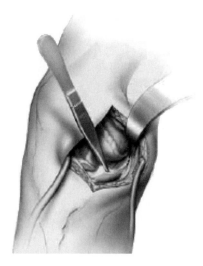

Fig. 6. Median parapatellar incision with view of the medial femoral condyle and tibial plateau.

femoral condyle. Osteophytes are also resected in a similar fashion along the medial border of the tibia. This resection creates pseudo-laxity of the medial collateral ligament and allows for complete restoration of the medial compartment joint space. Any osteophytes overhanging the medial border of the patella should also be resected, as they may impinge on the femoral sulcus when the femoral tibial axis is corrected from varus to valgus.

The next portion of the procedure includes a chondroplasty of the femoral condyle and tibial plateau. This procedure is done with power rasps to create a smooth gliding surface along the femur and the tibia (Fig. 7). This smooth gliding surface is necessary to allow a smooth, kinematics motion of the mobile UniSpacer within the medial joint compartment.

Care should be taken to balance the flexion and extension gap using these power rasps. One area of special attention is the area at the lowest end of the femoral sulcus just above the femoral notch. Cartilage just above the notch must be removed to allow the

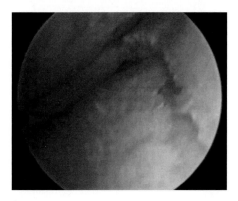

Fig. 5. Arthroscopic view of the medial compartment of a knee demonstrating full-thickness loss of articular cartilage on the tibia and femur.

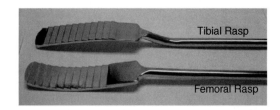

Tibial Rasp

Femoral Rasp

Fig. 7. Rasps used to contour the femoral condyle and tibial plateau.

anterior lateral flange of the device to nest into this region during full extension. Fig. 8 demonstrates the resulting impingement when this most important step is omitted.

Sizing of the device is for length and thickness. The device comes in six different lengths, ranging from 38 mm to 58 mm. Thickness sizes vary from 2 mm of thickness to 5 mm of thickness in 1 mm increments. Instruments within the set allow the surgeon to take preliminary measurements for length and thickness, but final sizing is determined after trials are implanted into the medial compartment. The goal of the trialing is to select the correct size, which fills the gap in the medial compartment to effect the proper axis correction from varus to valgus. Care should be taken to retension the medial collateral ligament and ACL. Overstuffing the medial compartment will lead to stiffness, specifically in the form of flexion contractures. Underfilling the medial compartment will lead to laxity of the ligaments and potential dislocation of the device. Although the proper length of the device is initially sized off of the tibia, the final length measurement is ultimately determined by the best fit to the femoral condyle radius.

Undersizing the implant will lead to edge loading of the device anteriorly and posteriorly, and eventual erosion of the remaining articular cartilage, whereas oversizing the device will lead to excessive overhang off of the tibial plateau and soft tissue impingement. The final best fit is determined by the visual inspection of the kinematics of the UniSpacer trial in addition to fluoroscopic confirmation in the AP and lateral planes.

Because the device is a mobile-bearing shim, it should follow the femoral condyle through normal rollback during flexion and extension. The device will have a normal anterior excursion in extension and a normal posterior excursion in flexion as the

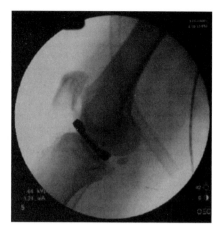
Fig. 9. Lateral radiograph of the knee demonstrating anterior excursion of the implant in extension.

femoral condyle rolls posteriorly. The device will also demonstrate rotation with the femoral axis between flexion and extension (Figs. 9 and 10). Once the final size is confirmed visually and fluoroscopically, final implantation of the UniSpacer is performed. The wound is then closed in layers with heavy, nonabsorbable sutures in the medial retinaculum, and absorbable sutures in the subcutaneous tissue. The use of drains or pain pumps can be used according to the surgeon's preference.

Routine antibiotic prophylaxis is used for 24 hours, and deep vein thrombosis (DVT) prophylaxis can be used according to the surgeon's preference, based on the patient's specific risk factors. Physical therapy initially focuses on range of motion, especially extension, and regaining quadriceps

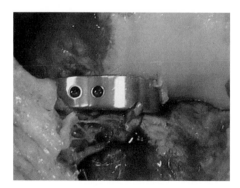
Fig. 8. Photograph of the knee with anterior impingement of the UniSpacer on the femoral condyle.

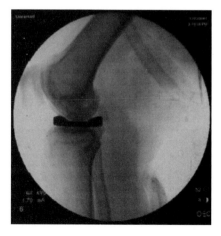
Fig. 10. Lateral radiograph of the knee demonstrating posterior motion of the implant as the knee flexes.

strength. Open chain exercises in the form of quadriceps setting exercises, straight leg lifts, and knee extensions allow the patient to regain strength without putting undue irritation on the biologic surfaces remaining in the medial compartment that articulate with the UniSpacer.

Postoperative management

Postoperative management is different from the typical management of a low-friction arthroplasty. The surgery may be performed as an inpatient procedure with a typical one-night hospital stay or as an outpatient procedure. The arthrotomy and debridement performed with this procedure do produce moderate postoperative pain. Femoral nerve blocks are helpful in controlling this pain. In addition, outpatients are best treated with an intra-articular pain pump. Inpatients may use a patient controlled analgesia (PCA) pump at the bedside. Pain management at home ultimately continues with oral analgesics.

DVT prophylaxis is again an individualized decision. Routine prophylaxis can range from aspirin (ASA) to low molecular weight heparin to coumadin. That choice is based on surgeon preference and patient risk factors. For instance, a surgeon may use ASA routinely, but may choose low molecular weight heparin for the patient who has a history of DVT, pulmonary embolism (PE), or chronic venous stasis. Duration of prophylaxis is again based on surgeon preference and patient risk factors.

Patients are given routine antibiotic prophylaxis during induction of anesthesia. Outpatients are given a second dose of parenteral antibiotics before discharge from the outpatient unit followed by 24 hours of oral antibiotics. Inpatients are given parenteral antibiotics during their overnight hospitalization.

Each patient needs close postoperative supervision in the outpatient office/clinic setting. Routine visits are scheduled for 2 weeks, 6 weeks, 3 months, 6 months, and 1 year. These visits are necessary to monitor patient pain level, knee effusion, and rehabilitation progress. As previously stated, all patients have postoperative effusions. Small effusions will gradually subside without intervention, but large effusions respond well to aspiration and injection with a cortisone product, which is best done, if necessary, at the 6-week and 3-month evaluations. If a patient still has some discomfort at the 6-month visit, viscosupplementation can provide symptomatic relief. Patients need to be educated preoperatively about the length of the recovery process and the possibility of aspiration to relieve swelling. Most patients will have

rapid improvement over the first 3 months followed by gradual improvement over one full year. Patients who have a slower path to recovery will need support and encouragement from the physician and the physical therapist.

If range of motion is not improving by the 6-week evaluation, manipulation under anesthesia will provide an increase in range of motion and a reduction in pain. Manipulations are much softer than those for TKRs, and improvement following the manipulation is much quicker. Fluoroscopic evaluation of the motion of the implant through the arc of flexion and extension during the manipulation will rule out any mechanical dysfunction of the device. Injection with cortisone will greatly reduce postmanipulation irritation.

Routine radiographs are performed at regular intervals during the postoperative period to ensure proper positioning of the device. An AP-erect view of the knee should demonstrate a device with the anterior flange of the device rotated toward the intercondylar notch. This view ensures that the device is following the normal convergence of the femoral condyles in the weight-bearing extended position. A lateral erect and flexion radiograph will demonstrate anterior translation in the extended position and posterior translation in the flexed position. Any deviation from these normal patterns must be correlated with the patient's clinical course.

Clinical results

Pain relief and improvement in clinical function are presumed to be related to correction of axial alignment and restoration of ligament balance. An average correction of 5° in the femoral tibial axis has been achieved in two groups of patients. The results of two subsequent sets of patients have been compared with respect to conversion and revision rates and clinical outcomes as defined by Lysholm scores, Knee Society scores (KSS), Knee Society function scores, and levels of satisfaction. The follow-up period is between 15 and 48 months.

Methods

The results from the first 79 knees (Group 1) are compared with the next 78 knees (Group 2). A surgical revision is defined as revision of one hemiarthroplasty implant to another hemiarthroplasty implant. A surgical conversion is defined as conversion implant to a TKR.

Results

In Group 1, 69 knees (87%) still had a UniSpacer after an average 33 months follow-up (range 30–48 months). At 24 months, 95% of Group 1 reported being happy. In Group 2, 74 knees (95%) still had a UniSpacer after an average 23 months follow-up (range 15–30 months). At 12 months, 97% of Group 2 reported being happy. The revision rate in Group 1 is 10% (8 knees) compared with a revision rate of 0% (0 knees) in Group 2. The conversion rate (UniSpacer to TKR) dropped from 13% (10 knees) in Group 1 to 5% (4 knees) in Group 2. The femoral tibial angle was corrected an average of 5° in Group 1 and an average of 4.5° in Group 2. Clinical scores in Group 1 improved an average of 38 points in Lysholm, 49 points in KSS, and 22 points in Knee Society function score. Clinical scores in Group 2 improved an average of 25 points in Lysholm, 40 points in KSS, and 11 points in Knee Society function score. At 12 months, 97% of Group 2 reported being happy. The revision rate and conversion rate dropped significantly between Group 1 and Group 2. The dramatically improved revision rate (UniSpacer to another UniSpacer) reflects improvements in surgical technique. The improved conversion rate (UniSpacer to TKR) reflects refinements in patient selection. The efficacy of the device has also been evaluated with respect to age of the patient and body mass index (BMI). Knee Society function scores (Table 1) definitely show a decline in improvement when comparing patients younger than 45 years to patients older than 65 years. Lysholm scores show similar trends, but the results are less dramatic. The device should not be used in patients over the age of 65 years (Tables 1 and 2).

The average BMI of the first 100 patients was 32. The results of two groups of patients were compared. Patients who had a BMI of less than 32 had an average BMI of 27. Patients who had a BMI more than 32 had an average BMI of 37. The results of the KSS and Lysholm were nearly identical, showing no decline in heavier patients (Table 3).

Table 1
Chart of Knee Society scores stratified by age

KSS function	Preoperative	>1 year postoperative
<45 years	64.00	82.14
45–54 years	56.08	75.27
55–64 years	58.15	72.92
≥65 years	52.35	61.94

Table 2
Chart of Lysholm scores stratified by age

Lysholm	Preoperative	>1 year preoperative
<45 years	41.86	76.79
45–54 years	47.22	74.97
55–64 years	40.07	79.69
≥65 years	48.18	77.06

Results demonstrate that significant obesity is not a contraindication for the use of the UniSpacer.

Complications

Complications for UniSpacer surgery can be categorized as generic lower extremity surgical complications and specific UniSpacer complications. Virtually any knee arthroscopy or arthrotomy procedure carries with it the potential risk for either an infection or deep vein thrombosis/pulmonary embolus. The surgical technique itself does not pose any other additional risk over and above what would be expected from similar procedures. Antibiotic and DVT prophylaxis are recommended preoperatively and continued postoperatively. Patients who have an extraordinary risk for either of these two complications may require a customized treatment program specific to their needs.

In addition to generic complications, the procedure also carries the risk for complications specific to UniSpacer surgery. Anterior dislocation of the device, residual postoperative pain, and arthrofibrosis can result from errors in patient selection and errors in surgical technique. Selection errors would obviously include performing surgery on contraindicated patients who have bone defects, ACL/PCL ligament deficiencies, flexion contractures, and far-too-advanced disease. Proper surgical technique requires proper sizing and site preparation. Implants that are too short or too thin are predisposed to dislocation; implants that are too long or too thick are predisposed to postoperative pain and stiffness (Fig. 11).

All patients have some effusion during the postoperative period. An aggressive chondroplasty or

Table 3
Results by body mass index

	Number	BMI	Lysholm	KS score	KS function
BMI 24–month data	37	<33	44–83	31–79	54–82
Average 33 months	31	≥33	42–80	27–79	57–73

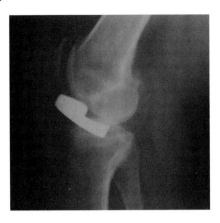

Fig. 11. Lateral radiograph showing dislocation of the UniSpacer.

sculpting of the femoral condyle and tibial plateau to match the femoral and tibial surfaces of the UniSpacer will reduce these effusions and facilitate a quicker recovery. The more congruent the surfaces are at the time of surgery, the quicker the recovery time.

Summary

The UniSpacer is a mobile-bearing shim that corrects axial alignment by an average of 5°. It demonstrates stable kinematics clinically and in laboratory testing. Femoral rollback is maintained throughout the arc of motion. Clinical results have significantly improved as the surgical technique has evolved and improved with instrumentation, specifically the power rasps. Complication/revision rates have decreased with the refinement of the surgical technique and patient indications/contraindications. The UniSpacer demonstrates the best clinical results in younger patients who have significant pain and functional disability. Obesity is not a contraindication and does not adversely affect the clinical outcome. It may be used as a good bridge procedure in younger patients because it does not alter the patient's bony or ligamentous anatomy.

References

[1] Emerson Jr RH, Potter TA. The use of McKeever metallic hemiarthroplasty for unicompartmental arthritis. J Bone Joint Surg Am 1985;67(2):208–12.
[2] MacIntosh DL, Hunter GA. The use of the hemiarthroplasty prosthesis for advanced osteoarthritis and rheumatoid arthritis of the knee. J Bone Joint Surg Br 1972;54(2):244–55.
[3] Scott RD, Joyce MJ, Ewald FC, et al. McKeever metallic hemiarthroplasty of the knee in unicompartmental degenerative arthritis. J Bone Joint Surg Am 1985;67(2):203–7.

ELSEVIER
SAUNDERS

Orthop Clin N Am 36 (2005) 513 – 522

ORTHOPEDIC
CLINICS
OF NORTH AMERICA

Unicompartmental Knee Replacement

Jack M. Bert, MD[a,b,*]

[a]Summit Orthopedics, Ltd., 17 West Exchange Street, Suite 307, St. Paul, MN 55102, USA
[b]University of Minnesota School of Medicine, Minneapolis, MN 55102, USA

Hemiarthroplasty of the knee, first described in the 1950s, refers to the concept of placing a spacer in one half of the femoral tibial joint to prevent bone on bone apposition. McKeever [1] first introduced his Vitallium (Zimmer Inc., Warsaw, IN) tibial plateau (Fig. 1) in 1957. MacIntosh [2] followed with an acrylic tibial plateau (Fig. 2) in 1958, and then one made of Vitallium in 1964. MacIntosh and colleagues [3] then presented their initial series in Switzerland in 1967 and published findings from a series of patients in 1972 that demonstrated "good results" in most patients who had follow-ups of 6 years [2]. The modern-day version of the hemiarthroplasty is the Unispacer (Smith & Nephew, Inc., Memphis, TN) (Fig. 3A, B), with results from 2-year follow-ups reported as 80% successful [4].

In the early 1970s, the Gunston and polycentric unicompartmental knee arthroplasties were introduced (Fig. 4A, B). The revision rate of these early devices at 2 years was approximately 10% [5,6]. Multiple authors from 1973 to 1983 noted success rates varying between 37% and 92% with 2- to 8-year follow-ups [5–13]. From 1987 to 1991, long-term results were published with 87% to 90% survivorship at 13 to 16 years [14–16].

From 1990 to 1993, several authors reported 90% to 96% fair to good results using a combination of metal-backed and all polyethylene tibial components with 2- to 7-year follow-ups [17–21]. These reports were the first to note that obese patients had a 1.4 times greater failure rate [18].

Multiple survivorship studies were reported from 1993 to 2003, with success rates from 87% to 98% with 6- to 14-year follow-ups [22–30]. In one series, 83% of the failures were caused by progressive wear in the unresurfaced compartment [27].

Because of the resurgence in popularity of unicompartmental knee arthroplasty (UKA), primarily as a result of the mini-incision technique [30], it is important to understand the advantages and disadvantages of this procedure compared with total knee arthroplasty (TKA) and upper tibial osteotomy (UTO), and the indications and contraindications for this procedure.

When comparing UKA with TKA, 75% of the patients who had UKA in one knee and TKA in the other note that their UKA "feels closer to a normal knee" than their contralateral TKA (Fig. 5). The UKA knee had better range of motion and decreased blood loss compared with TKA [31–33]. In addition, because only one third of the knee joint is being replaced, the biomechanics of a UKA are closer to a normal knee than are those of a TKA [17].

When comparing UKA with UTO (Fig. 6), the results of UKA in three different series were significantly superior with 3.5- to 15-year follow-ups. In these studies, there were 46%, 48%, and 65% success rates for UTO compared with 76%, 90%, and 88% for UKA, respectively [34–36].

The advantage of UKA is that it allows for preservation of bone stock, improved range of motion, reduced blood loss, reduced inpatient stay, and decreased cost. In a community-based hospital registry in St. Paul, Minnesota, a review of 240 UKA cases with a 15-year follow-up showed a mean range of motion of 127°, mean blood loss of 350 mL, and a mean length of stay of 2.8 days

---

* Summit Orthopedics, Ltd., 17 West Exchange Street, Suite 307, St. Paul, MN 55102.
E-mail address: bertx001@tc.umn.edu

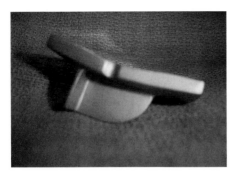

Fig. 1. McKeever hemiarthroplasty prosthesis.

(compared with 5200 TKA cases that had a mean length of stay of 4.5 days) [37]. UKA is easy to revise [38] if excessive amounts of bone have not been removed (Fig. 7A, B). However, in two published series with 7- to 10-year follow-ups, only 75% to 85% of patients had good to excellent results [39,40]. In these two studies, up to 75% of the patients had significant osseous defects (Fig. 8A, B). In a personal series of 31 cases that had a mean follow-up of 9.2 years, 96.3% had good to excellent results but only 4% of these cases had significant osseous defects [41]. Furthermore, a study of 47 revision UKAs from a community-based registry in St. Paul, with a follow-up from 1.9 to 16 years and a mean follow-up of 9.4 years demonstrated a 94% survivorship (Jack M. Bert, submitted for publication, 2004). Additionally, Lewold [42] noted in 1998 that conversion to TKA after UKA is easier and more successful than conversion from UTO to TKA.

The disadvantages of UKA include poor instrumentation and design [43], uncemented systems failures [40], and poor fixation. The design of the undersurface macrostructure of the tibial component in UKA is critical to its ability to withstand shear and offset loading in the laboratory [44,45]. A reduced survivorship has been reported compared with TKA, with development of arthritis in contralateral compartment (Fig. 9) resulting in early failure [26,27,29].

The clinical indications for UKA are that the patient should have a sedentary occupation, there should be less than 10° of varus deformity, range of motion should be at least 90° without a flexion contracture, there should be medial instability only, the patient should not be obese, the diagnosis should be osteoarthritis (OA) or posttraumatic arthritis, and most importantly that there should be unicompartmental pain only [43]. To clinically assess unicompartmental pain, the patient should have a positive

"one finger test" (Fig. 10). This test is performed by having the patient point to the involved compartment with one finger when asked to locate their pain. This is in contradistinction to the patient who performs a "knee grab" when asked to locate their pain (ie, the patient can't localize their pain to one area in their knee and literally grabs the entire knee when asked to locate their pain) (Fig. 11). When this knee grab occurs, a TKA rather than a UKA should be performed. Therefore, UKA should not be performed on everyone who has strictly unicompartmental disease if the remainder of the knee is symptomatic. In fact, when three different active knee surgeons were asked to determine which patients who had OA of the knee they considered to be appropriate candidates for UKA, Stern and colleagues [46] reported only 6%, Bramby and colleagues [47] reported 15%, and Laskin [48] reported 12%. Commonly accepted roentgenographic indications [49] for UKA are 50% unicompartmental joint space collapse (Ahlback I) and complete collapse (Ahlback II) on standing radiograph views (Fig. 12A, B).

Because of improvements in survivorship studies of UKA as a result of improvements in prosthetic devices and surgical technique, UKA should be considered in two additional patient categories. The first group is the middle-aged OA patient who desires a reliable initial result with retention of both cruciates and easy revision to TKA if necessary. The second group of potential candidates is geriatric patients who are not likely to survive the lifespan of the UKA and may have medical problems precluding a major reconstructive procedure such as a TKA [50]. UKA in this last patient group may improve the patient's lifestyle and reduce a significant amount of the patient's ambulatory and rest pain.

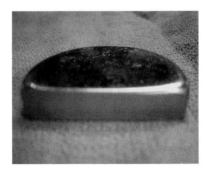

Fig. 2. MacIntosh hemiarthroplasty prosthesis.

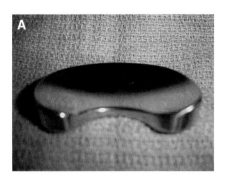
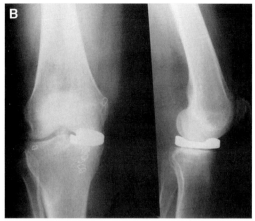

Fig. 3. (*A*) Unispacer component. (*B*) Anteroposterior and lateral postoperative x-ray.

Contraindications to UKA are rheumatoid arthritis, nonlocalized knee pain, decreased range of motion with a flexion contracture, active lifestyle (sports), obesity, knee instability with absence of the anterior cruciate ligament (ACL), and unrealistic expectations regarding the activity level and longevity of the prosthesis. Young heavy laborers must be educated regarding the limitations of a UKA and this type of patient may be better served by an osteotomy. Radiograph contraindications are grade IV Ahlback changes (Fig. 13) consisting of joint space obliteration plus medial-lateral subluxation of 3 to 4 mm. Operative contraindications consist of moderately

significant bi- or tricompartmental disease, contralateral grade IV Outerbridge [51] changes on the femoral or tibial weight-bearing surfaces (Fig. 14), an absent ACL, and greater than 10° of varus deformity for medial compartment disease. An absent ACL usually indicates more significant contralateral compartment changes precluding UKA. Patellofemoral disease is not a contraindication to UKA unless the patient had preoperative patellofemoral symptoms [22,52].

Failures of UKA have many causes. In a series of 31 failed UKA cases published in 1997 [41], 35% had medial-lateral mismatch (Fig. 15), 19%

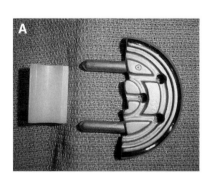
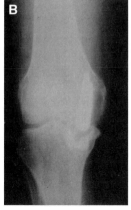

Fig. 4. (*A*) Polycentric components. (*B*) Anteroposterior postoperative x-ray.

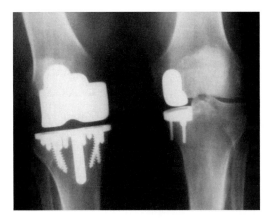

Fig. 5. TKA and contralateral UKA in same patient.

laterally to facilitate what is often a difficult exposure. Two self-retaining retractors are then used to help expose the medial compartment. An external tibial cutting jig is applied to the leg and no more than 4 to 5 mm of bone is removed from the tibia. Bone should be removed laterally to the insertion of the ACL. The tibial cut surface must be perpendicular to the shaft of the tibia and most systems allow for 3° to 5° of posterior inclination of the tibial component. The femoral surface is measured with a sizing device and a cutting jig is applied to the femur. After cutting, burring, or rasping the surface down to cancellous bone (depending on the system that is being used), the trial femoral component is fit to the joint surface, the fin slots are burred if necessary, and the femoral peg hole is drilled to accept the femoral component. Regardless of which component and instrumentation system are used, the femoral component should always be lateralized on the femur to avoid medial-lateral mismatch during extension and flexion. Femoral components that are too small or narrow if medialized tend to maltrack and may sublux during extension, especially if a smaller, narrower tibial component is chosen for implantation. After preparing the bony cut surfaces with multiple drill holes and drying, as has been recommended for TKA [53], the components should be cemented simultaneously, checked for appropriate tracking throughout flexion and extension, and the knee then placed in full extension as the cement hardens. Care must be taken to make certain that all cement is removed from the joint despite the limited exposure afforded by this

had failed uncemented ingrowth (Fig. 16), 16% had malaligned tibial components (Fig. 17), 10% had failed cemented femoral components (Fig. 18), 10% had failed tibial polyethylene component wear (Fig. 19), and 10% had progressive, contralateral compartment OA (Fig. 9). Refinements in UKA component design have occurred over the past 30 years. It is important to have articulating geometry that avoids increased surface-contact stresses. The articular surfaces between the components should have the ability to allow for minor variations in medial and lateral placement of the components and afford the ability to accept a minor difference in rotational malalignment during flexion and extension of the knee. Thus, the component articular surfaces cannot be severely constrained nor should they be flat on flat. Furthermore, it is imperative to use a system with a wide femoral component that will obviate medial-lateral mismatch [50]. Finally, it is important during placement of the prosthesis that the instrumentation used does not require significant resection of either femoral or tibial bone. If significant bone resection occurs, revision arthroplasty will be difficult [39,40].

The minimally invasive limited incision surgical technique involves approximately a 6- to 10-cm medial incision (Fig. 20) for a medial compartment UKA extending from 1.5 cm inferior to the joint line approximately 5 to 6 cm superiorly along the medial edge of the patella. Incising superiorly into more than 5 to 6 mm of the vastus medialis insertion should be avoided if possible. The medial compartment is exposed and a quarter-inch Steinman pin is drilled into the intercondylar notch to retract the patella

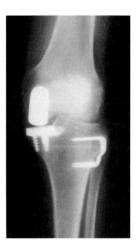

Fig. 6. UTO followed by UKA in the same patient.

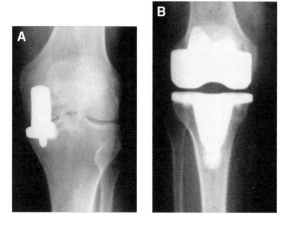

Fig. 7. (*A*) Painful UKA. (*B*) Postoperative revision TKA.

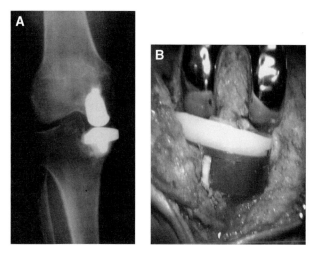

Fig. 8. (*A*) Painful UKA with marked tibial bone loss. (*B*) Revision TKA with wedge augmentation.

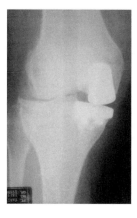

Fig. 9. Progression of arthritis in contralateral femoral tibial compartment.

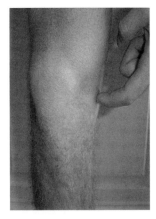

Fig. 10. One finger test.

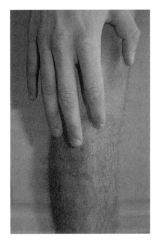

Fig. 11. Knee grab.

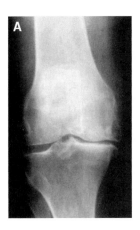
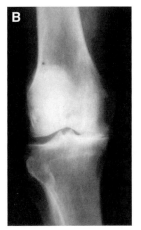

Fig. 12. (*A*) Grade I Ahlback changes (50% joint space collapse). (*B*) Grade II Ahlback changes (complete joint space collapse).

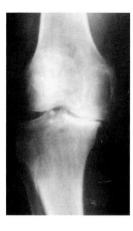

Fig. 13. Grade IV Ahlback changes with medial-lateral subluxation.

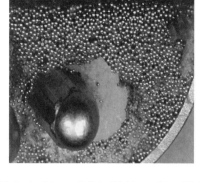

Fig. 16. Lack of ingrowth into tibial base plate with failure of fixation.

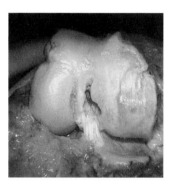

Fig. 14. Grade IV Outerbridge changes on the lateral femoral condyle with "kissing lesion" indicating medial lateral instability.

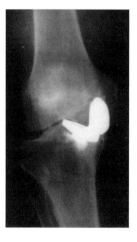

Fig. 17. Malaligned tibial component.

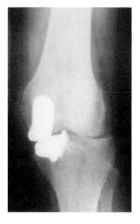

Fig. 15. Medial-lateral mismatch of femoral and tibial components.

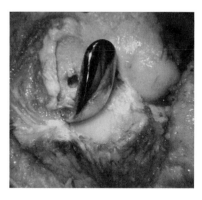

Fig. 18. Failed cemented femoral component.

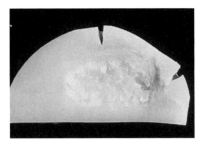

Fig. 19. Failed tibial polyethylene component wear.

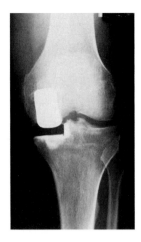

Fig. 21. Postoperative view of well-positioned cemented UKA.

technique. A hemovac drain should be placed before fascial and skin closure and a soft dressing placed. Most patients are discharged 24 to 48 hours after this procedure and must use a cane for the first 2 weeks (Fig. 21).

Unicompartmental arthroplasty is a successful procedure in a moderately active older patient who has strictly unicompartmental pain and understands that the prosthesis is not going to last forever. It is a reasonable procedure to perform in the elderly patient who is unable to medically tolerate a TKA. Limited incision techniques work well with appropriate instrumentation. The selected prosthetic device should be based on logical design principles and tested biomechanical rationale. A UKA is still simply a UKA despite newer techniques of implantation, better instrumentation, and updated prosthetic devices. The indications for this procedure are significantly different and separate from those of a TKA.

The single most important factor for the success of this operation and the most difficult to ascertain is appropriate patient selection. A well-performed

UKA implanted in the wrong patient will definitely eventually fail!

References

[1] McKeever DC. Tibial plateau prosthesis. Clin Orthop 1960;18:86–95.
[2] MacIntosh DL, Hunter GA. The use of the hemiarthroplasty prosthesis for advanced osteoarthritis and rheumatoid arthritis of the knee. J Bone Joint Surg Br 1972;54:244–55.
[3] MacIntosh DL. Arthroplasty of the knee in rheumatoid arthritis using the hemiarthroplasty prosthesis. In: Stuttgart GC, editor. Synovectomy and Arthroplasty in rheumatoid arthritis; second international symposium. Stuttgart, Germany: Theime; 1967. p. 79.
[4] Friedman MJ. UniSpacer. Arthroscopy 2003;19(10): 120–1.
[5] Skolnick M, Peterson LF, Combs JJ. Polycentric knee arthroplasty. A two-year follow-up study. J Bone Joint Surg 1975;57A:1033.
[6] Skolnick M, Coventry M, Ilstrup D. Geometric total knee arthroplasty. A two-year follow-up study. J Bone Joint Surg Am 1976;58A:749–53.
[7] Bae D, Guhl J, Keane S. Unicompartmental knee arthroplasty for single compartment disease. Clinical experience with an average four-year follow-up study. Clin Orthop 1983;176:233–8.
[8] Laskin RS. Unicompartmental tibiofemoral resurfacing arthroplasty. J Bone Joint Surg Am 1978;60:182–5.
[9] Cameron HU, Hunter GA, Welsh RP, et al. Unicompartmental knee replacement. Clin Orthop 1981;160: 109–13.
[10] Insall J, Aglietti P. A five to seven-year follow-up of

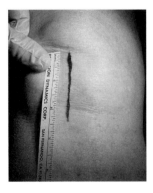

Fig. 20. Minimally invasive UKA incision.

unicondylar arthroplasty. J Bone Joint Surg Am 1980; 62:1329–37.

[11] Insall J, Walker P. Unicondylar knee replacement. Clin Orthop 1976;120:83–5.

[12] Marmor L. The modular knee. Clin Orthop 1973; 94:242–8.

[13] Marmor L. Results of single compartment arthroplasty with acrylic cement fixation. A minimum follow-up of two years. Clin Orthop 1977;122:181–8.

[14] Marmor L. Unicompartmental arthroplasty of the knee with a minimum ten-year follow-up period. Clin Orthop 1988;228:171–7.

[15] Scott RD, Cobb AG, McQueary FG, et al. Unicompartmental knee arthroplasty. Eight- to 12-year follow-up evaluation with survivorship analysis. Clin Orthop 1991;271:96–100.

[16] Rand JA, Ilstrup DM. Survivorship analysis of total knee arthroplasty. Cumulative rates of survival of 9200 total knee arthroplasties. J Bone Joint Surg Am 1991;73:397–409.

[17] Hodge WA, Chandler HP. Unicompartmental knee replacement: a comparison of constrained and unconstrained designs. J Bone Joint Surg Am 1992;74: 877–83.

[18] Heck DA, Marmor L, Gibson A, et al. Unicompartmental knee arthroplasty. A multicenter investigation with long-term follow-up evaluation. Clin Orthop 1993; 286:154–9.

[19] Cobb AG, Kozinn SC, Scott RD. Unicondylar or total knee replacement: the patient's preference. J Bone Joint Surg Br 1990;72:166–95.

[20] Sisto DJ, Blazina ME, Heskiaoff D, et al. Unicompartmental arthroplasty for osteoarthrosis of the knee. Clin Orthop 1993;286:149–53.

[21] Rougraff BT, Heck DA, Gibson AE. A comparison of tricompartmental and unicompartmental arthroplasty for the treatment of gonarthrosis. Clin Orthop 1991; 273:157–64.

[22] Cartier A, Sanouiller JL, Grelsamer RP. Unicompartmental knee arthroplasty surgery. 10-year minimum follow-up period. J Arthroplasty 1996;11:782–8.

[23] Grelsamer R. Unicompartmental osteoarthritis of the knee. J Bone Joint Surg Am 1995;77:278–92.

[24] Kennedy W, White R. Unicompartmental total knee arthroplasty of the knee: postoperative alignment and its influence on overall results. Clin Orthop 1997;221: 278–85.

[25] Tabor Jr OB, Tabor OB. Unicompartmental arthroplasty: a long-term follow-up study. J Arthroplasty 1998;13:373–9.

[26] Squire MW, Callaghan JJ, Goetz DD, et al. Unicompartmental knee replacements. A minimum 15 year follow-up study. Clin Orthop 1999;367:61–72.

[27] Bert J. 10-year survivorship of metal-backed, unicompartmental arthroplasty. J Arthroplasty 1998;13: 901–5.

[28] Svard UC, Price AJ. Oxford medial unicompartmental knee arthroplasty. A survival analysis of an independent series. J Bone Joint Surg Br 2001;83:191–4.

[29] Gioe TJ, Killeen KK, Hoeffel DP, et al. Analysis of unicompartmental arthroplasty in a community-based implant registry. Clin Orthop 2003;416:111–9.

[30] Repicci JA. Total knee or uni? Benefits and limitations of the unicondylar knee prosthesis. Orthopedics 2003; 26(3):274.

[31] Newman JH, Ackroyd CE, Shah NA. Unicompartmental or total knee replacement? Five-year results of a prospective, randomized trial of 102 osteoarthritic knee with unicompartmental arthritis. J Bone Joint Surg Br 1998;80:862–5.

[32] Laurencin CT, Zelicof SB, Scott RD, et al. Unicompartmental versus total knee arthroplasty in the same patient. A comparative study. Clin Orthop 1991;273: 151–6.

[33] Rougraff BT, Heck DA, Gibson AE. A comparison of tricompartmental and unicompartmental arthroplasty for the treatment of gonarthrosis. Clin Orthop 1991; 273:157–64.

[34] Karpman RR, Volz RG. Osteotomy versus unicompartmental prosthetic replacement in the treatment of unicompartmental arthritis of the knee. Orthopaedics 1982;5:989–92.

[35] Broughton NS, Newman JH, Baily RA. Unicompartmental replacement and high tibial osteotomy for osteoarthritis of the knee. J Bone Joint Surg 1986; 68:447–52.

[36] Weale AE, Newman JH. Unicompartmental arthroplasty and high tibial osteotomy for osteoarthrosis of the knee. A comparative study with 12- to 17-year follow-up period. Clin Orthop 1994;302:134–7.

[37] Bert J. Analysis of unicompartmental arthroplasty in a community based registry. Presented at American Academy of Orthopedic Surgeons. Dallas, February 13, 2002.

[38] McAuley JP, Engh GA, Ammeen DJ. Revision of failed unicompartmental knee arthroplasty. Clin Orthop 2001;392:279–82.

[39] Lai CH, Rand JA. Revision of failed unicompartmental total knee arthroplasty. Clin Orthop 1993;287: 193–201.

[40] Padgett DE, Stern SH, Insall JN. Revision total knee arthroplasty for failed unicompartmental replacement. J Bone Joint SurgAm 1991;73:186–90.

[41] Bert J, Smith R. Failures of metal-backed unicompartmental arthroplasty. Jrnl Knee 1997;4:41.

[42] Lewold L. Revision of unicompartmental knee arthroplasty. Acta Orthop Scand 1998;69:469–74.

[43] Bert JM. Universal intramedullary instrumentation for unicompartmental knee arthroplasty. Clin Orthop 1991; 271:79–87.

[44] Bert JM, Koeneman JD. A comparison of the mechanical stability of various unicompartmental tibial components. Orthopedics 1994;17(6):559–63.

[45] Rosa RA, Bert JM, Bruce W, et al. An evaluation of all-ultra-high molecular weight polyethylene unicompartmental tibial component cement fixation mechanisms. J Bone Joint Surg Am 2002;84A(Supp 2):102–4.

[46] Stern SH, Becker MW, Insall JN. Unicondylar knee

arthroplasty. An evaluation of selection criteria. Clin Orthop 1993;286:143–8.

[47] Bramby S, Thornhill T. Unicompartmental osteoarthrosis of the knee. In: Laskin RS, editor. Controversies in total knee replacement. London: Oxford University Press; 2001. p. 285.

[48] Laskin RS. Unicompartmental knee replacement: some unanswered questions. Clin Orthop 2001;392:267–71.

[49] Ahlback S. Osteoarthrosis of the knee: a radiographic investigation [thesis]. Stockholm, Sweden: Karolinskca Institute; 1968.

[50] Scott R. Unicompartmental total knee arthroplasty.

In: Insall JN, Scott WN, editors. Surgery of the knee, Vol. 1. Philadelphia: Churchill Livingston; 2001. p. 1621.

[51] Outerbridge RE. The etiology of chondromalacia of the patellae. J Bone Joint Surg Br 1961;43B:752–7.

[52] Corpe RS, Engh GA. A quantitative assessment of degenerative changes acceptable in the unoperated compartment of knees undergoing unicompartmental replacement. Orthopedics 1990;13:319–23.

[53] Bert J, McShane M. Is it necessary to cement the tibial stem in cemented total knee arthroplasty? Clin Orthop 1998;356:73–8.

ELSEVIER
SAUNDERS

Orthop Clin N Am 36 (2005) 523–533

ORTHOPEDIC
CLINICS
OF NORTH AMERICA

Cumulative Index 2005

Note: Page numbers of article titles are in **boldface** type.

A

Abrasion arthroplasty, in articular cartilage defect repair, 419–420

Acetabular component fixation, 129
hip resurfacing arthroplasty and, 190–191

Acetabular fixation, cemented *vs.* cementless, 105–107

Acetaminophen, for unicompartmental arthritis of knee, 403

Acrylic bone cements
acetabular revisions with, 81
alternate bearing surfaces with, 80
antibiotic(s) and, 24–26
antibiotic prophylaxis with, 55–56
application of
current status in Japan, 86
technique for, 86–87
as alternative to bone cement, Manchester symposium on, proceedings of, **105–111.** See also *Bone cement, acrylic bone cement alternatives to, Manchester symposium on, proceedings of.*
aseptic loosening with, mechanism of, 76–77
bone loss and, 83
clinical development of, **85–88**
in North America, **75–83**
complications of, 85–86
composition of, **17–28**
creep behavior with, 34–35
curing of, 18–21
current status of
in Japan, **85–88**
annual total sales, 85
in North America, **75–83**
development of, 3
after 1960, 6–9
dislocations due to, 82
early experience with, 75–76
failure with, definition of, 76
fatigue behavior with, 35–38

fatigue failure with, 6
femoral design issues with, 77–79
femoral revisions with, 80
functions of, 17
future of, 59
general concepts related to, 81–83
genesis of, 2–3
handling properties of, 21–23
heat formation of, 18–21
in Scandinavia, **55–61**
infections due to, 81–82
liquid components of, 17–18
mechanical properties of, **29–39**
static, 29
mechanism of, 76–77
molecular weight of, 26–27
physical properties of, **29–39**
powder components of, 17–18
problems associated with, 83
properties of, **17–28**
radical polymerization of, 18–21
radiopacity of, 26
residual monomer and monomer release with, 23–24
static mechanical test methods, 31–32
according to ISO 5833, 29–31
sterilization of, 26–27
surgical approach to, 82–83
technique for, 56–59, 80–81
thromboembolic issues related to, 82
types of, 55–56
viscosity of, 21–23
volume shrinkage of, 18–21
water uptake and glass transition in, 32–34
wear of, 79–80

Adjacent level degeneration, reduction of, 234–235

Allograft(s)
articular cartilage, 462–463. See also *Articular cartilage allografts.*
disease transmission risk and, 460
history of, 459–461